THE FAILED BACK SURGERY SYNDROME

J. ANTONIO ALDRETE

CORPUS

THE FAILED BACK SURGERY SYNDROME
Jorge Antonio Aldrete
1st Edition

Aldrete, Jorge Antonio – The Failed Back Surgery Syndrome
Jorge Antonio Aldrete – 1ª ed. – Rosario
Corpus editorial y distribuidora, 2006
62 p.; 24x16,5 cm

ISBN 950-9030-19-8

1. Medicina-Síndrome Quirúrgico. I. Título

CDD 616.87

editorial@corpuslibros.com.ar
aldrete@corpuslibros.com.ar
www.corpuslibros.com.ar
Suipacha 581 – Tel/Fax (+54 341) 439 4978
(S2000AOB) Rosario – Argentina

Editor: Esteban Oscar Mestre

Esta tirada se terminó de imprimir
en Talleres Gráficos Fervil S.R.L. Santa Fe 3316 Tel.: 0341 437 2505
E-mail: fervilsrl@arnet.com.ar • 2000 Rosario • Santa Fe • Argentina

This edition was printed in march 2006
Rosario – Argentina

Author

J. ANTONIO ALDRETE MD, MS

Professor, Department of Anesthesiology
University of Alabama at Birmingham
Birmingham, Alabama

Aldrete Pain Care Center, Inc., Birmingham, Alabama
Sunshine Medical Center, Inc., Chipley, Fl

Contents

Preface

Among other attributes, I have been called by some "Champion of Unpopular Causes" and by others "Proponent of Unwanted Ideas"; be that as it may, in the past I:

- Participated in the pioneer team of surgeon Tom Starzl and defended vigorously, liver transplantation, at the time in the 1960's and 70's, when it appeared to some, to be an unethical and hopeless idea, because there was a low long term survival rate[1].
- With the assistant of Diane Kroulik, proposed and insisted that all patients having surgery be objectively evaluated, as they recovered from surgery and anesthesia and developed the Post Anesthetic Recovery Score. Although rejected by an editor as "it has no clinical relevance" it has become the standard of care as a criteria for discharging patients from Recovery Rooms[2].
- With Harry Lowe and Bob Virtue published the first book and organized the first Congress on Low Flow and Closed System anesthesia technique, advocating the development of equipment (flowmeters, ventilators and vaporizers) that would allow to use minimal flows, when the use of high flows of gases was the norm[3].
- Along with Frank Guerra, we called attention to the need to consider the psychological aspects of patients having surgery and anesthesia, at the time when no one admitted all the attention was directed to getting the patient well without considering the fears, anxiety and depression that patients may exhibit before and/or after surgery[4,5].
- In the pre-manged care era (1980's), together with other collaborators, we analyzed the cost of anesthetic equipment, gases and other drugs, comparing the expense derived from the various anesthetic techniques popular at the time[6].
- Derived from personal experience with patients with chronic pain, attention was given to one more untold and unpopular cause, when in the year 2000, the publication of the first book pointing out that Arachnoiditis, a disease no one wanted to hear about, was becoming an epidemic[7].

Now just when hardware used for spinal fusions is producing exorbitant financial gains for manufacturers, implanters and all others involved, I dare to point out that this enormous expense placed on the health care systems is not only not helping many patients, but it is harming some of them driving up the disability rate, which many of them are reaching at a premature age.

In the past, physicians who have dared to call attention to harmful trends in Medicine have been castigated by our peers; this punishment has ranged from isolation, de-certification, vilification and financial ruin. I do not mind a fair debate or controversy since Medicine is hardly an exact science.

However, this book blames no one but a system that has developed on its own, ensuing of terrible outcomes; most importantly, it is a call for re-rapprochement to traumatic and degenerative diseases of that wonderfully built organ, the spine. It belongs to several specialties including Neurosurgery, Orthopedics, Neurology, Physiatry, Anesthesiology, Psychiatry, Radiology, Psychology and Pain Medicine specialists who in one way or another care for patients given the ominous diagnosis of "Failed Back Surgery Syndrome".

To write this book, I have not only reviewed thousands of pertinent publications, although for the sake of brevity, only those that appeared pertinent to the points discussed were included; this by no means, implies that those references not cited were irrelevant, only that it was intended to avoid repetition. There are seven tables and four photographs of patients, but as readers will notice, there are no drawings in this treatise. It is the opinion of the author that must drawings included in books do not actually represent the actual anatomical reality of patients with spinal medical conditions. Instead, as diagnosis and to guide treatment more than thirty radiological images have been used to represent precisely the examples intended to guide the readers who are urged to not only read the radiologist report, but also to become familiar with the images representing pseudoarthrosis, clumped nerve roots, impingement of a nerve root, spinal cord compression, spinal stenosis and also to learn to differentiate a disk bulge from a protrusion or a herniation and to identify osteophytes wherever they may be located, as they may also be "pain generators". Finally, I would like to propose that the indications for whatever procedure to be done in these patients be clearly stipulated and discussed with the patients; they are to be used mostly as therapeutic modalities and not as diagnostic methods, as all of them (differential spinals, discography, sympathetic blocks) may have risks. Myelography followed by a CAT scan is only indicated when MRI is contraindicated, otherwise it has been shown to be an exacerbating factor in patients with inflammatory spinal diseases.

This compendium is dedicated to the many patients that have received this diagnosis, which most of them have never heard of before and even when they think they understand it, they do not realize the actual life ahead of them. By making it available to all health care practitioners it is intended to present a different point of view that has in the past been given. Emphasis was placed in the reliability or the lack of it, of certain diagnostic tests used to identify the several conditions present in their spine and related structures. Of great importance is avoiding the procedures that may lead to this disabling disease.

In my opinion, the prognosis of FBSS is guarded, not because of its lethality but because of its lack of effective and long lasting treatment, making it sore of dismal as chronic, unrelented pain, medication dependency, serious physical disability and psychological disturbances drastically deteriorate the patients quality of life. At best, as of 2006, the only trully effective measure against it is prevention. That means doing only procedures that have shown to be beneficial to these patients by a meta-analysis and supported by objective evidence, as recommended in the last portion of the book.

J. Antonio Aldrete, MD, MS

Introduction

1

Those that might have read the first edition of the "Arachnoiditis: the silent epidemic" book may wonder if this is a sequence to it and why the different focus toward the failed back surgery syndrome (FBSS). This is not a follow-up, but the readers deserve an explanation. From the time I began taking care of patients with this insidious disease, in 1989, I have noticed certain trends; in general and rounding numbers, initially, about 40% of patients had began to experience symptoms suggestive of arachnoiditis (ARC) after a pantopaque myelogram, though frequently, they went on to have spinal surgery, too. There were also, about an equal number (30%) of patients that had developed ARC after spinal surgery and others that developed it after having pain relief procedures before or after having had surgery.

Obviously, the numbers of patients whose disease started after myelograms, by attrition have dwindled, after 1986 when pantopaque was removed from the market. The few cases that I see these days caused by myelography are remnants from that era. Both the medical community and the public are more aware of the feasibility of developing ARC from complications of some of the spinal injections, as well as from spinal and epidural anesthesia. Adjustments have been made on those therapeutic modalities and on the use of neuraxial anesthesia in efforts to reduce such morbidity. However, of late, the majority of patients seen in our clinics have acquired arachnoiditis from either laminectomies, and especially, from spinal fusions performed mostly with hardware. Of notice is the publication of a landmark article by Deyo et al [1] in the New England Journal of Medicine entitled "Spinal Fusions: a case for restraint" which showed a considerable rise of this type of operation pointing out to the lack of sustainable evidence that they improve the outcomes of patients with low back pain , while unquestionably increasing their disability, increasing the number of surgical operations and augmenting the cost of their care, substantially [2,3].

Strong commercial forces encourage the use of hardware to replace elements of the remarkably well built organ, the human spine, that is made to support us in the erect posture for longer and longer periods as longevity is in the rise and we are expected to do more physical activities designed to keep physical fitness, though demanding greater wear and tear of the spine.

From these trends, in the last two decades, a relatively new descriptive diagnosis, has been coined labeling it the "Failed Back Surgery Syndrome (FBSS)", also entitled "Failed Back Syndrome", when surgery was not involved; it appears to me that this denomination has been given to more and more patients, every day[4]. The rationale for this nomenclature is not evident but it seems to be related to patients with an unspecific diagnosis of "low back pain" who after having had one or more operations and many more interventions in the spine, their initial complaints appear to have been made worse, rather than improved, reaching a point where no further operation is feasible or indicated. The apparent representation appears to be that the trend is to perform a series of treatment modalities, over a period of two to six years, if not improved, then the patients are given again an ultra, non-specific diagnosis suggesting that the patients' back, failed to get better. This unfair terminology essentially avoids having to list one by one, every diagnosis that patients end up with, after numerous and sometimes repeated therapeutic attempts failed to alleviate their initial symptomatology.

In reality no one wishes or dares to tell the patient, through out his calvary, that the pain he/she has can be managed conservatively, up to a point and the possibility that some of these interventions, specifically, after operations of the spine, sometimes the pain may be worse, the neurological deficit greater, so the disability will be substantial.

It is not clear whether this terminology was formulated to identify a new category of disease entity (including spinal surgery), or to avoid having to specifically mention some of the added complications that may reveal the failure of the treatment given (including spinal surgery). It seems that from lack of a better global term that would list all the diagnosis and almost "by default", FBSS has been incorporated to the medical jargon[5] and amazingly, also into the medical code books[6]. In a way, this attribute is not fair to the patients because as a negative term, they do not understand it; moreover, it casts a stigma that assumes that there is nothing else positive that can be done to help them and what is worse, they may be considered abusers of the health care system and not uncommonly they are prejudicially treated as drug seekers. Somehow it seems that most of them, in their journey of sorrow, end up in pain management facilities as they no longer fit into any of the conventional specialty clinics and their condition has failed to progress, as expected. The fact is that the most common diagnosis given to them at the onset of their disease was "Low Back Pain", a non-specific diagnosis that allows first-care givers to treat all of them the same[7] regardless of their clinical signs and symptoms and at the opposite end of their disappointing course they are again assigned a non-specific diagnosis. "Failed Back Surgery Syndrome".

There are few systematic reviews of randomized controlled trials of patient outcomes after the first-time laminectomy[2,3,6], nevertheless, there are numerous protocols including rehabilitation, physical fitness, exercises and others that are aimed to have the patient return to work and to readjust to the new reality as a post-laminectomy patient. Undoubtedly after these operations patients have certain fears such as re-injury, re-herniation or instability of the spine. Ostello et al[8] were able to accept only 13, out of hundreds of studies reviewed, that would satisfy the requirements of the Cochrane Controlled trials. Patients that recovered more promptly and returned to their physical activities were those that took up intensive exercise programs that were started within 4 to 6 weeks after surgery, versus more moderate training protocols. Although none of the treatments given produced harm to the recovery of the patients, neither supervised training, multidisciplinary rehabilitation, low-tech and high-tech exercises, physical agents and joint manipulations made any significant improvement in the physical recovery of the patients studied.

In reality each case varies from one to the next, though the majority of patients have one or more common denominators that appeared after one of the spinal operations or one of the invasive interventions, as well. These may include:

- Recurrent Disk Herniation
- Peridural Scarring
- Nerve Root Compressed by Scarring
- Deformity of the Dural Sac
- Herniation of an Adjacent Disk
- Spinal Instability
- Facetectomy
- Pseudomeningocele
- Arachnoid Cysts
- Arachnoiditis
- Foraminal Re-stenosis

Not uncommonly after portions of discs are removed and laminectomies are extended laterally, the spine becomes "destabilized" as the facet joints have been rendered dysfunctional and painful. The sequence follows with a spinal fusion indicated supposedly to stabilize that portion of the spine. Although spinal fusions suppose to convert two or more vertebrae into one bony unit, with or without hardware, they may result in one or more of the following:

- Pseudoarthrosis
- Malposition of Screws
- Protrusion of Screws through the Vertebral Body
- Protrusion of Screws into the Vertebral Canal (Figure 1)
- Fracture of Screws
- Loosening of the screws
- Displacement of Hardware (cages)
- Intrathecal Scarring
- Intrathecal Calcification (Figure 2)
- Impingement of Nerve Roots
- Pedicular Pain
- Paravertebral Muscle Dysfunction and Atrophy

Historical perspective

To best understand this syndrome, a brief historical description of the events that brought about the circumstances, now in play, is in order. Invasive entry into the neuraxis was initiated by Quincke[2] in 1885, when he performed the first lumbar puncture to sample the cerebrospinal fluid. Attempts to visualize the contents of the dural sac were led by Dandy[10] in 1919 who injected air into the subarachnoid space in patients that resulted in the advent of pneumomyelography producing only a borderline radiographic visualization of the spinal cord and nerve roots. Myelography was introduced in 1922 by Sicard and Forrestier[11] by injecting lipiodol (iodized poppy seed oil) intrathecally and took plain roentgenograms that allowed them to have a fair visualization of the spinal contents; however because its high viscosity and low miscibility with the CSF, it was discarded. Eventually dyes with lower density, but almost as toxic, such as Abrodil, Thorium oxide, and Kontrast[12] were tried but all showed poor definition of images and frequent complications[13]. Meanwhile, Mixter and Barr[14], in 1934, defined lumbar herniated discs as the main cause of sciatica; it was then that disk excision, through a laminectomy, initiated the trend for elective surgical operations of the spine. This was facilitated by the introduction of ethyliodophenyl undecylate (Pantopaque), which was first administered to patients in 1944, providing a good definition and contrast of images, establishing myelography as the standard test to identify spinal pathology[15]. Because it was the contrast media of choice pantopaque was used extensively in spite of multiple reports of arachnoiditis[16,17,18]. After laminectomies, spinal fusions were proposed for correction of scoliosis and traumatic injuries; initially they were done with bone graft and lately with metal hardware. These procedures have given the impression that extensive interventions of the spine were feasible and uneventful.

Rationalization for spinal surgery

2

Though the removal of a compressive lesion from a tubular osseous structure containing delicate neural elements such as the spinal cord, nerve roots, dural sac and cerebrospinal fluid (CSF), more often than not, eliminates the pain and dramatically improves the affected function (s); however, surgical access into the spine does not occur without risks and consequences.

Zeidman and Long[19] defined this syndrome as "the condition resulting from one or more surgical interventions, with disastrous results with persistence of back pain and exacerbation of the pre-existing complaints, characterized by a constellation of symptoms, that include referred pain to the lower extremities, sphincter dysfunction, physical impairment and psychological alterations associated with diseases of the spine." What has not been clarified is the fact that patients seek medical attention, requesting help for pain in their back; whatever procedure performed with this purpose that does not relief the back pain, ought to be considered a failure.

This fact is pertinent to laminectomies and especially to spinal fusions even when a solid arthrodesis is achieved; however if the patient's pain continues, in reality, they have not succeeded. It is evident that, the objectives of these spinal operations need to be redefined directing their aims to only utilize therapeutic modalities that have proven to effectively relief the specific pain experienced by that specific patient[7,20]. Moreover, modalities such as microdiscectomies have not proven to be safer or less expensive nor do they have a lower morbidity[4,5,21,22].

Laminectomies

As far as epidemiology, it is not possible to know exactly how many of these operations are performed in the US, annually. Franklin et al[20] noted that after correction for differences in population, Americans have operations on their spine (laminectomies and fusions), eight times more than citizens of other industrialized countries. Considering that low back pain is one of the most prevalent diseases of middle and older age, the cost for these interventions is considerable when approximate calculations have suggested that more that 900 000 spinal operations are performed annually in the United States[23] (considering that some patients may be operated more than once in one year's time); however, when gross estimates[1,2,4,19] have figured that from 15 to 30% of these cases ultimately may end up with the diagnoses of FBSS, these calculations are staggering. Since there is a life time incidence of back pain in about 80% in the general population, these numbers are substantial, because by the time the diagnosis of FBSS is reached, it is estimated that, on the average, more than 250 000 US dlls. have already been spent on the care of those patients. Not knowingly, at that point, their predicament is that they contemplate disability, rejection, persistent pain and suffering for the remainder of their life time[24].

The reasons for the disparity in the frequency of indications for surgery of the spine among industrialized countries are numerous[25], but the most relevant are as follows:

- Greater labor protection given to workers in other industrialized countries, where lifting pulling and carrying, in industries, hospitals and construction is done mechanically by pulleys and lifters, permanently installed and strategically placed, rather than by humans, to avoid back injuries
- Back saving education is a subject taught in schools and is taken seriously by supervisors, students and workers, alike.
- The financial incentive is undoubtedly an uncontrollable factor that influences excessive surgical intervention in the private practice of medicine versus conservative therapy in institutional or socialized medicine. The need to establish rigorous criteria for the indication of these surgical interventions of the spine is obvious as this approach[4,26] and other interventionism[27,28] have been shown to be extremely expensive while no compelling proof has been demonstrated that a definite cure is certain for this common ailment[29].
- Lack of specific clinical guidelines as to when and what operations are indicated for each specific condition that produces low back pain.
- The inadequate control that governmental agencies exercise over new surgical procedures, and the implantation of medical devices[30].
- Lack of implementation of evidence-based medicine as a necessary proof that new treatments truly benefit patients approving them only after comparative, impartial, double blind, control studies have been performed[31].
- The ultimate proof that a procedure or an operation relieved the patient's pain would be to accept the recently proposed "result based medicine" in which payment is only obtained if the outcome is favorable.

Most, if not all, of these cases start with low back pain; after a variable degree of conservative therapy, they are offered a laminectomy to remove the herniated portion of a disk supposedly because the corresponding nerve root is compressed by such herniation. The usual manifestations include symptoms and signs of radiculopathy. The most common access into the spinal canal is through the posterior approach usually requiring a laminectomy or a laminotomy. Even then, access to the degenerated disk is narrow and frequently complicated by swelling of the affected nerve root that has been compressed[32]. This may improve soon thereafter, but in some cases the distal end of the root can actually become more swollen[33], depending on the radicular vascular response to surgical manipulation (either traction or pressure on the nerve roots), while being released[34].

The consequences from a laminectomy have to be considered individually accepting that the main objective is the relief of the low back pain that motivated patients to seek help[26]. It is obviously apparent that the outcomes in patients under 30, having one single degenerated intervertebral disk are more favorable than in middle age individuals with 2 or 3 affected discs and some degree of spondylosis, especially in smokers[35]. The outcomes are less hopeful in elderly patients that have multiple levels and degrees of disk disease, facet joint arthritis, osteoporosis (Figure 2), pseudoarthrosis and spinal stenosis. However, because of work related injuries, motor vehicle accidents and possibly other factors, the middle age group, proportionally, undergoes spinal surgery more often[5,20,36].

In his classic treatise, Wilkinson[4] admitted that "the conclusion that in America many failed back syndromes result from excessive surgical intervention seems difficult to avoid". He listed the following supporting reasons:

- Incorrect Diagnosis that may include misdiagnosed neoplasms, the so called "flabby back syndrome" common in affluent societies where obesity is prevalent, rheumatoid arthritis, osteoarthritis, osteoporosis, ankylosing spondylitis, etc.[23,35]. Not uncommonly, patients may have symptoms of radiculopathy in one lower extremity, though the radiological findings are located on the opposite side; to operate on the side of the symptoms may ensue in disastrous outcome, since the pathology is where the radiologist described it[36].

- Unnecessary Surgery, such as operating on a bulging disk, without radiculopathy symptoms; slight sensory loss does not necessarily mandate operation. To perform fusions in grade I spondylolysthesis is still under debate[2].
- Improper or Inadequate Surgery; such as disk excision performed at the wrong level, the wrong side, leaving a loose fragment of disk or selection of the wrong hardware to secure a fusion[4,37].

To these surgeon-dependent factors, at least three more types of predisposing factors may be added:

- The presence of short pedicles, lumbarization of S1 (figure 3), sacralization of L5 and arachnoid cysts.
- Inadequate imaging or inconclusive interpretation may offer misleading diagnosis or fail to recognize associated pathology such as vertebral hemangiomas and scoliosis, stenosis, absence of peridural space. The diagnostic value of invasive tests such as differential blocks, epidurography, discography, etc. is very much in doubt, as most pathology can be identified by a carefully and detailed interpretation of an MRI[38]. Provocative procedures performed by injecting dyes or local anesthetics, have come under scrutiny as they are usually performed by the person who will interpret them and that will carry on the next procedure. For example, in discography 1.0 ml of dye produces little pain in normal and ruptured discs alike, but if 2.5 ml of dye are injected in normal, bulging, protruding or herniated discs, pain will be elicited at every level injected, casting doubt on this procedure (Figure 4). Moreover, to inject the dye, the puncture with a large size caliber needle (18 or 16 gauge) may weaken the annulus fibrosus of a previously normal disc[39].
- CAT scans or three dimensional tomography, are non-invasive but provide limited information as the dural sac contents can not be identified; whenever possible, MRI is to be used, with contrast, to better determine the cause of the recurrent pain.
- Not to be considered lightly are the economical forces that favor equipment manufacturers, hospitals, physicians and associated groups to perform procedures with undefined outcomes.

On the other hand, there are a number of measures that patients can take for themselves, to improve their own outcomes; for example,

- Stop cigarette smoking; this habit has been found to decrease the threshold of pain[39], increase perioperative narcotic requirements[40], affect wound healing[41], increase postoperative pulmonary morbidity[42] and add to the patients stress response[43]. Furthermore, it increases dural sac pressure during bouts of coughing, facilitating CSF leaks[44]. Nevertheless, this issue is seldom discussed between doctors and patients; as a matter of fact, some consider this habit a relative contraindication to proceed with surgery in patients that refuse to stop smoking. Since most of these operations are not done in emergency basis, postponement of the operation for two to three months will definitely reduce postoperative pulmonary morbidity and improve outcomes considerably.
- Obesity is frequently encountered in middle age patients, the most common

age group having spinal surgery. There is no hard evidence however, that loosing weight might decrease low back pain, but it certainly improves health, in general and allows for easier physical activity. Moreover, there is no question that caring for the patient with morbid obesity, presents greater difficulty for all doctors and nurses, every procedure is more difficult, there is higher incidence of respiratory complications, wound infections, deep venous thrombosis and pulmonary emboli. Preferably, loosing weight should be done before, rather than after the operation.

- Lack of having a program destined to improve the patients' physical fitness even before surgery, followed by a more active, but not prematurely forced physical therapy program that includes aquatherapy and the rational use of orthotics (figure 5).

Indications for spinal fusions

As perplexing as it may sound, spinal fusions are in some cases the cause of FBSS and in some instances they are the effect necessary to try to resolve certain cases of the same syndrome. This apparent paradox can best be explained by accepting the fact that in no instance is there a deliberate intent to harm a patient, but only the hope that by forming one bone out of two or three, the patient's pain and other related symptoms will be relieved. Unfortunately, more often than not we are not willing to admit that this is wishful thinking. As new devices are being brought to the market, we have seen promotions repeating themselves, first there were the Steffee plates (Figures 4, 6, 7) and screws[30] that have been approved by the FDA only for long bone use[45] received with great enthusiasm, only to find out that the screws often fractured or became loose six months later, leaving the patients in greater disability and pain. The metal initially used was stainless steel, that was replaced by titanium, at a much greater cost, but soon it was noted that these latter metal screws, two years later, became disengaged from the pedicle also leaving a trace of microscopic residue that elicits a chronic inflammatory reaction[45,46].

The intended objective is to construct a fixed single unit out of two movable vertebral bodies and still be the magnificent weight bearing structure built by nature with the laminae and the spinous process while protecting the neural elements contained in the vertebral canal (Figure 7). The degeneration of the spinal units usually occurs slowly due to repeated minor trauma and the aging process, both of which can be accelerated by heavy loads such as in construction workers, truck drivers, porters and athletes that participate in contact sports. Undoubtedly, the multiple spinal units are morphologically designed to stand pressure load while linked by ligaments and supported by muscles but limited flexion, extension and rotation[47].

Four stages of degeneration

Stage I: is characterized by the loss of water from the gelatinous disk that may appear in films as a "vacuum phenomenon", also identified by a loss of intervertebral space height.

Stage II: is noted by changes in the chemistry and physiology of the disk noted as accumulation and decline in cell nutrition resulting in decreased concentration of viable cells, cell senescence and degraded matrix molecules.

Stage III: is typified by an increase in the spinal segment motion, producing symptoms of instability as a result of posttranslational modifications of collagen, decrease water content and compromised cellular function.

Stage IV: by then the unit develops progressive fatigue failure unable to readjust morphologically to demands of repetitive deformation. Then osteophytes form from a continuous process of calcification leading to stiffness within the spinal segment and in some instances bridge two vertebrae, laterally, essentially a natural fusion process.

Attempts to replace intervertebral discs

After describing the unique structure and function of natural discs, when they undergo a degenerative process and especially after partial removal of the degenerated (herniated) portion of the disk at laminectomies, the options are a second discectomy or a fusion with bone graft in between the vertebral bodies or a disk replacement. The latter has been more popular in the last decade as fusions with screws and plates have failed so badly. Interbody fusion cages received great promotion, a campaign that eventually showed the lack of benefit when compared to placebo[47]. The enthusiasm for replacing discs, first with metal cages, expected bone grafts placed within, to stimulate new bone graft. It was not only difficult to perform, but frequently the cages were displaced and occasionally compressed the adjacent nerve roots (figure 8). After numerous failures with cages, following extensive sophisticated research, various models of movable disk replacement [48] have been introduced without satisfying the most simple of requirements of medical evidence[49]; the series have included few patients, the following-up period has been relatively short and the extraperitoneal approach to implant them has been plagued with potential complications to other organs leave a great to be desired. The posterior approach is cumbersome and potentially hazardous to neural structures (dural sac and nerve roots).

Other probable complications may be resorption of bone graft, more likely to occur when movement of the fused-junction occurs soon after the fusion had been performed, leading to painful pseudoarthrosis[50]. When soft tissue (fat or muscle) is present between the bone fragments, it will prevent proper fusion by impeding the adherence of bone fragments to each other. Painful pseudojoints (Figure 8) usually result in back pain, when standing or walking, without radiculopathy; however if osteophytes or hypertrophic scar tissue develop beneath the the pseudoarthrotic line, it may extend into the epidural space producing traction or compression of nerve roots manifested by sciatica type of pain[51].

Overgrowth of the bone fusion may produce a painful "kissing" pseudoarthrosis when both bone surfaces become in direct contact (Figure 8). If located proximal to the vertebral canal, it may also result in spinal stenosis that may compress the dural sac and the elements within, usually manifested by neurogenic claudication characterized by diffuse aching pain in the legs, aggravated by walking and continuing, even if the walking stops (contrary to claudication that occurs in vascular insufficiency).

Resorption of bone results from the opposite process with gradual dissolution of the implanted bone graft material, whether autologous or homologous. It may be complicated by wound infection and occasionally osteomyelitis, requiring aggressive antibiotic therapy and rarely drainage and removal of the loose fragments. In any of the above mentioned possible complications, pain relief may be obtained by thoraco-lumbar-sacral bracing, specially adjusted to each individual patient that usually would give stability to the lower spine (Figure 5). Diagnosis of the condition of the fusion can be confirmed by plain roentgenograms, testing it in flexion and extension and CAT scans; stenosis of the canal may be revealed by 3-Dimensional CAT scan (Figure 6) or MRI (Figure 1).

The criticism of the rapid rise of spinal operations in general and fusions in particular questions the aggressive promotion approach used by seductive technological advances but undefined indications, which in some cases have been fostered by financial incentives to the parties involved, all of whom have derived greater revenues[1,49,50], only to discard their previous device when a new idea enters the market. This may be a good sales strategy, but in this case, the defective or malfunctioning apparatus was left inside of patients' spines. This market has been estimated to exceed 2 billion U.S. dlls a year and with an annual growth of 20%. Other innovations, including spinal fixation devices, computer-guided and minimally invasive surgeries, placebo surgery, as well as other supplements such bone-graft substitutes and morpho-genetic proteins, have had some popularity but have provided little evidence of efficacy. They have potential for high reimbursement without hard data found in the published studies[5,30,50].

Some reports[52,53], included as few as 14 patients, followed for short intervals have overstated the safety and efficacy of these procedures leading to the over-utilization of a technology still in question that may lead to unnecessary invasive procedures that could aggravate the patients pain and disability with a diagnosis of Failed Back Surgery Syndrome.

As Deyo et al[1,2], and Wilkinson[4,36] have strongly cautioned, the enthusiasm for new technology, associated with high rates of use, but unproven acceptable outcomes must be tempered, because of the high rate of failures and morbidity. Replacing totally the intervertebral discs, not only has not shown sufficient favorable results that can be accepted[48,54,55], but when total disk arthroplasty fails and has to be removed, it leaves the two adjacent plates of the vertebrae in direct contact, without any cartilaginous cushion, essentially leaving one bone resting on the one below, an anti-anatomical, unstable joint with heavy contact and extreme load (Figure 8) that elicits continuous pain.

3 What fails in the 'Failed Back surgery syndrome'

The answers are multiple, and since at any one time, one or more of these complications may cause the reappearance of pain and neurological deficits after these operations. In addition of the predisposing factors already mentioned, the duration of the patient's pain, whether there has been or not pain-free intervals, work capabilities, as well as, the psychosocial history of each individual patient-candidate[29],[31], all have to be considered. The following causes provide some explanation, though they are not listed in order of frequency or seriousness of their occurrence:

Poor selection of patients

It has been suggested as the most common cause of FBSS, since the main complaint of the patients is pain, the decision to perform a laminectomy at one or two levels, to do a foraminotomy or a facetectomy would have to be based not only on the physical and radiological findings, but also on the real possibilities of eliminating, that patient's pain. If the whole cause of the patients' symptoms is a herniated disk pressing on a nerve root the results would most likely be satisfactory[36]. But if in addition there is a grade I spondylolisthesis, spondylosis, or spinal stenosis, the possibility of completely relieving the pain is unlikely[19,22]. However, the reality is that if such patients are deterred from surgery, even when an appropriate explanation is given to them, it is feasible that some will continue to "doctor-shop" until they find a surgeon willing to operate, assuring them that the result "is going to be fine". This quagmire has no real solution as long as the system does not work in unison, applying the same indications for the same lesions and having the same aims, for all patients[2,56]. The fact is that in some cases, such as central and paracentral protruding or herniated discs, of less than 4 mm extension into the vertebral canal, may be treated conservatively, unless they become larger or wider producing significant radiculopathy[57].

Incidental durotomy

Perhaps, one of the most underrated complications, nevertheless, it may occur in 6 to 8% of first time laminectomies, 12 to 20% in repeat laminectomies and in 14 to 30% of the spinal fusions[58,59]. Recognition of these tears allows them to be repaired on site promptly. Unrecognized tears not only would result in CSF leak, but also would allow for blood to accumulate at the bottom of the wound (in patients in the prone position) and therefore to enter the subarachnoid space[60]. This usually unexpected development may have serious consequences as blood is an active irritant of nerve tissue and may initiate an arachnoiditic inflammatory response. Depending of the amount of CSF lost, postural headache and even meningismus may occur in the immediate postoperative period, especially if there is a bulging mass under the incision, or worse if cerebrospinal fluid leaks through it, in which case it may be tested for sugar content with a glucose strip. Ultimate confirmation can be obtained by an MRI of the lumbar spine (figure 9). If CSF is present in the retrospinal tissues, eventually a soft, thin pseudo-sac will form (Figure 10) that contains it. If not initially repaired, this membrane will give rise to a pseudomeningocele or an enlargement and deformity of the dural sac[60] (Figure 1). Puncture is not recommended as CSF may leak, persistently[61]. Attempts to stop the leak by draining the fluid continuously for several days by inserting an intrathecal catheter, have low chances for success and may produce infection or a subdural bleed[22].

A review of 146 medical malpractice cases conducted by Goodkin and Laska[60], in patients undergoing lumbar spine surgery, had an incidence of 15.7% (23 cases) of unintended, "incidental durotomy" (ID), which was the second most frequent occurrence. In every case, there was an associated complication or long-term sequelae; therefore ID should be considered a most serious event. CSF leaking through the wound was a warning sign in six cases (23%), a pseudomeningocele formed in five (21.7%) of them, cauda equina syndrome was diagnosed in 11 patients (43.4%) with uni- or bilateral foot drop in 8 of these cases (34%). All these instances are indeed catastrophic neurological deficits that resulted in poor outcomes and in no way should be taken lightly [21,61].

Recognized or unrecognized, dural sac entry may also be accompanied by nerve root contusion and/or trapping giving rise to the so called "Battered nerve root syndrome" [19,26]; cauda equina manipulation, leaving foreign materials (instruments, sutures, gelfoam, thrombin glue, etc) have both been incriminated in producing ARC when applied to the dura[61,62,63,64,65], in addition allowing the passage of blood into the subarachnoid space, with its subsequent deleterious effects. Other surgical adverse events such as herniation of rootlets through the dural tear, expose them to ischemia and possibly to certain chemicals that may be applied extradurally. In addition, the tethering of roots (Figure 11) may increase tension during certain physical activities or when patients acquire certain positions like extreme flexion, turn from side to side or raise their legs, patients experience pain[61].

Discussion on the subject of causation of pseudomeningoceles, as well as, the various forms and differences between dural sac dilatation, ectasia, pseudo sac and dural cuff cysts, as well as the pros and cons of doing an earlier or a late repair and the chances for spontaneous resolution is beyond the scope of this chapter. Suffice it to say that peridural scarring, dural sac deformities and deviations (Figure 12) from its usual position, commonly seen in postoperative imaging studies, may place undue traction on the nerve roots, aggravating the symptoms of recurrent radiculopathy and manifesting as spinal stenosis, too.

Loose disk fragments

With an incidence from 2 to 7%, loose disk fragments of nucleus pulposus may be "drag out" of the annulus fibrosus cavity by the grand-jeurs instrument employed to remove the loose portions of the disc[21,22]. Less commonly, loose fragments can also come out of the nucleus pulposus cavity later on, days later, when the patient is mobilized. As the loose fragment is trapped in between the extradural, intracanal segment of the nerve roots, it begins to produce sharp, severe radicular pain, localized to the dermatome corresponding to the compressed nerve root that is being pressured by the 0.5 to 1.4 cm fibrocartilaginous mass (Figure 13). Confirmation is done with an MRI, requiring immediate surgical re-intervention as the patients are in severe constant pain and may also have a cauda equinoid syndrome[66,67].

Intrathecal and or peridural hematoma

Either are serious events. Substantial amount of blood in the subarachnoid space is manifested by severe, burning low back pain with or without radicular symptoms appearing immediately upon patient's awakening from the anesthetic [62]. It usually requires considerable dosages of opiates to control it. More common are extradural hematomas (Figure 14), which initially present as moderate to severe low back pain but with moderate to severe paravertebral muscle spasm. Depending on the size of the hematoma and its proximity to the dural sac, back pain, neurological symptoms may appear two or three weeks postoperative, this may result from the degradation of blood elements and products and the subsequent liberation of leukotrienes and cytokines that are able to cross the dural barrier [68].

Nerve root cysts

Leg pain with minimal back pain, may be caused by postoperative cystic out pouchings when dural tears occur in the dural cuff that accompany the emerging nerve roots (Figure 15) during their intraspinal canal passage. They should be differentiated from the congenital arachnoid cysts (Figure 3) that occur at the same location. At myelography[69], they fill immediately. Postoperative arachnoidal cysts are formed at the time of surgery when a small dural tear occurs in this same sheath location, and if not corrected; the arachnoid that herniates through this dural tear, forms the primary cyst and is usually reinforced by an outer wall of fibrous tissue[58]. They may be identified by fluid pulsations. In any case, at surgery, the ostium or opening communicating with the subarachnoid space is very small and difficult to find[4,61]. Surgical repair may consist of invagination of the cyst, reinforcing the suture line then suturing the external dural wall, reinforcing it with a patch of fascia.

Epidural fibrosis

Is perhaps the most dreadful of complications from spinal surgery and the most frequent cause of FBSS[4,14]. Most laminectomies are usually followed by a short period (3 to 6 months) of improvement as the excision of the herniated portion of the disk, the removal of a portion of the lamina and the ligamentum flavum provide relief from the constrictive compression with a satisfactory result as the patients' symptoms subside or markedly improve[32,33]. All along, as the wound heals, an inflammatory response is occurring around the dural sac and the paravertebral muscles; eventually, the cellular infiltrate gives way to collagen deposition that proliferates for months and the incision heals, as all tissues in every organ do with scar tissue, the operated intervertebral space heals with collagen and fibrous tissue leading to scarring in the peridural space (Figure 16), fibrous adhesions to the dura, nerve roots, bone, muscles and fascia, where surgery took place[62,68]. In some cases, this proliferation of fibrotic tissue and adhesions is exaggerated and eventually it may indent or compress the dural sac and even encircle a nerve root[33]. If foreign bodies (Surgicel, Gelfoam, gauze, cotton pads, etc.)[61,62] or glues (ADPL[70,71,72] natural materials[26], etc.) are left in the wound, or there has been a difficult, traumatic access, or a large extradural hematoma, this reaction may be accelerated. Fatal anaphylaxis has occurred after fibrin glue application[73]. Symptoms of radiculopathy may appear according to the nerve root affected. However; not uncommonly, all these materials may provoke more inflammation, resulting in greater fibrosis and scarring[74]. It is here where meticulous surgical technique makes a difference[75].

The gradual surrounding of a nerve root by scar tissue produces radicular pain and sensory disturbances as it elicits traction and compressive effects on the root[33]. It is difficult to make the differential diagnosis if a recurrent herniated disk is suspected; in this latter case, the nerve root is displaced[34,75,76]. Electrodiagnostic studies may indicate the apparent location of the radiculopathy and the extent of nerve root dysfunction; however, for a more conclusive diagnosis, MR imaging with the IV contrast gadolinium is necessary, in order to enhance the scar tissue by the transfer of the dye from the intravascular to the interstitial space compartments, as it would occur from inflammation or scarring [77,78,79]. Caution on the interpretation is advised as high dose contrast (0.3 mmol/kg) has been demonstrated to increase the conspicuity of the disc[80]. Repeated attempts by the local instillation of any chemical substance, including steroids or any other anti-inflammatory agent, to prevent peridural scarring have not met with success[72,74,81].

Insufficient decompression

This may occur more often when the position of the herniation of the disk is lateral or when decompressive attempts to eliminate within the lumen of the lateral foramina, osteophytes or even bone residues, which might have compressed the nerve root, fail[82,83]. Within the spinal canal, central stenosis may be due to a hypertrophic ligamentum flavum, short pedicles, a loose disk fragment or a herniated disk in which case, wider decompression, such as obtained from a bilateral laminotomy or lateral foraminectomy, may be necessary in order to gain ample access to the pain generator lesion[84,85]. Bilateral facetectomies are not favored as they certainly destabilize the spine and increase the back pain[86].

Residual, recurrent or adjacent herniated disk

An incompletely removed herniation, may be extruded again as the annulus fibrosus is usually left open, liberating a free fragment in the vertebral canal[66,67]. Single HNPs more frequently happen in young patients (Figure 17); while middle age and senior patients frequently have several lumbar discs in various degrees of degeneration[87]. When a herniated portion of the most degenerated disk is removed, the usual torch forces change and the protruding or slightly herniated discs may not be able to tolerate the new undue pressures applied while in the erect position or during flexion[46,88,89], so adjacent discs continue to degenerate in an accelerated process and soon another disk is fully ruptured producing radiculopathy[90], depending of its size (> 4 mm) especially if its location is lateral (Figure 18) or broad when the nerve root is more likely to be compressed. Then, the need for another laminectomy becomes apparent, as the same pathological process may repeat itself creating a "domino effect" [87,91].

Mechanical instability

Some of the pre-existent abnormalities that predispose to lumbo-sacral spine instability have already been named, however, for the sake of completion, they will be mentioned again; the most common is the sacralization of L5, lumbarization of S1 (Figure 3) and scoliosis from 5 to 15 degrees. Usually, these congenital variances can be recognized in sagittal views of MRI films[92]. Others non-congenital, but post-surgical are bilateral facetectomies, extensive bilateral laminotomies, and severe unilateral spondylosis destabilize the adjacent segments of the spine[90,93,94]. Disalignment of adjacent vertebrae may occur after extensive discectomy leading to spondylolisthesis[8,95]. Alteration of the usually even axial surface of each vertebrae, by either scoliosis, a degenerated disk, an osteophyte or one sided spondylosis may change the individual support given by each segment. In addition, an unstable spinal segment(s) prevents the normal dissipation of the load sharing, thus changing the distribution of stress forces through out the axial topography of each vertebra[89,96].

Depending on which lesion predominates, spinal stenosis, spondylolisthesis or ligament stretching may result reducing and morphologically changing the transverse diameter of the vertebral canal and/or the neuroforamen. During the aging process, these changes occur gradually; in severe trauma, some of them may appear suddenly. Discectomies, as helpful as they may be in reducing the compression of neural elements, under certain circumstances, they may affect the stability of the spine precipitating the need for a stabilizing fusion[46].

Pseudoarthrosis

After spinal fusions, it is essential to monitor the stability of the fused unit; however, the usual plain films on flexion and extension, only show extreme cause of instability[77,79,97]. To define if bone growth is taking place between vertebrae, either a CAT scan[98] or an MRI[99] would be required in order to determine if there are any vacuum phenomenon or spaces (Figure 20) in between where new bone growth should be[100,101]. In all fairness, a maximum of two years is suggested as a waiting period for a fusion to be successful. If no "bone-pockets" persist, most likely the pseudoarthrosis is permanent. If hardware was applied, then as long as the screws and plates are in place and not causing side effects, they can be left in. However if pain persists, and the screw head sites are tender or there is bending of the plate (Figure 19) or screw fracture they may have to be removed. Leaving an unstable spine, frequently results in worse pain than before the fusion as the discs usually had been removed[102]. Occasionally when bone fragments are placed in between the vertebral bodies, close to the posterior edge, growing graft bone eventually may protrude into the vertebral canal acting as osteophytes, impinging upon the dural sac[51]. Repeat fusions are usually less likely to succeed than the first attempt[4,100,103].

Relief of pain by external bracing (Figure 5) has been considered an indication for spinal fusion, but if there are any of the predisposing factors for failure, bracing may be considered more permanently as fusions may have few chances to succeed in these individuals. Failure to obtain relief with external bracing is an ominous sign.

Sometimes, to define the integrity of a supposedly fused bony mass is difficult, as the vertebrae loose their usual anatomical features; radioisotope scans may be helpful, but not all the time. Resorption of mass may be detected by plain A-P and lateral films or by MRI and less likely in CAT scan (Figure 21) so it would be hypertrophic bone protruding into the vertebral canal[51]. Debris from metal implants sometimes may be shown initiating a foreign body reaction[104].

A large scale prospective randomized study is going on in the US, comparing the clinical outcomes of patients having circumferential fusion versus disk replacement. Thus far, one of the eighteen groups participating in the project has reported preliminary results at six months post-surgery; Delamarter et al[105] found that mobility of the spine was greater and disability was reduced in a group of 60 patients treated with the artificial "ProDisc", as compared to patients treated by fusion. This time, pain assessment, using the visual analogue scale showed conflicting results at three and six months post-surgery, although in both groups the back pain had been reduced from the control measurement.

Failures after 20 months are usually revealed by excessive or abnormal movement of one vertebra on another and pain on the site, chiefly in patients that have also extensive laminectomies, with or without facetectomies that rendered the spine unstable. When at plain films, in flexion, the fusion translates more than 8° of the AP diameter of the vertebral body, or rotates more than 9%; then it is assumed that the fusion has failed[100,102].

Spondylolisthesis

The overriding of a vertebra over the posterior plate of the one below results in undue compression of the posterior end of the intervertebral disk, narrowing of the lateral foramen and possible impingement of the corresponding nerve root producing moderate constant pain that is exacerbated by standing and walking[89,96,100]. According to the degree of disparity of the alignment of the two vertebrae involved, it has been given four grades (I to IV)[77,78]. Only grade I may be treated with conservative measures; higher levels of deviation usually require surgical stability. It is desirable not only to fix (by fusion), the two adjacent vertebrae but to attempt to correct the misalignment in order to relief the pain, as well[76,94].

In a prospective randomized study conducted by Thomsen et al[107] comparing a group of 64 patients treated for spondylolisthesis grades I or II to a group of 66 non-instrumented patients, with similar illness, showed that posterolateral fusion, with pedicles screw fixation, increased the operation time, the blood loss and re-operation rate, leading to a significant risk of neural injury. There was however, an improvement in the functional outcome, in the instrumented group. The authors concluded that there was no justification for the use of pedicle screw fixation alone, as an adjunct to posterolateral lumbar fusion.

Although spondylolisthesis can be seen in the first set of films in some patients seeking medical care for their low back pain (Figure 22), if the negative odds added by this condition are not recognized, the outcome of most interventions will most likely be in disadvantage, needed repeated intervention, re-operation and eventually a fusion that would be less likely to succeed than in a non-complicated spine[49]. This sequence of events, not only demonstrates poor diagnosis, but may eventually increase significantly the cost to the health care system and would render the performance of a fusion more difficult because of the scarring and fibrosis at the various intervertebral levels to be operated on[6,20].

Infections

Can occur in the soft tissues as cellulitis or fascitis (Figure 23), as an epidural abscess (Figure 24), or as meningitis with delayed clinical manifestations for up to one month[109]. Discitis may also be present producing localized pain, low grade fever, and malaise for months[21,110]. Ultrasound and/or radiological imaging[111] usually may identify the type, extent and location of the more superficial infections (Figure 24). If significant dural sac compression is evident or in case of signs of sphincter dysfunction, surgical exploration and abundant irrigation are mandatory[36]. However, most of them can be treated conservatively[112] with antibiotics, mainly those that cross the blood/brain barrier, analgesics, muscle relaxants and bed rest; however if neurological deficit persists, surgical drainage and evacuation may be necessary[109].

Sometimes, infections may be introduced into the intervertebral space and spread into the adjacent vertebral bodies resulting in osteomyelitis; they may be favored by the presence of residual hematoma, pseudomeningocele, necrotic tissue or free small disk or bone fragments that may be conducive to bacterial proliferation[103]. They may manifest first, only as moderate low back pain, low grade fever and general malaise[113]. Some authors[74,108,114] have noted a higher incidence of infections if the microscope is used over the open wound during surgery; however the usefulness of the apparatus usually out weights the risk of its use, nevertheless, it emphasizes the need for the most strict sterile technique, at all times.

Spinal stenosis

Repeated operations may produce both axial and radicular pain that may be caused by a herniated disk, hypertrophy of the facet joints (Figure 25) or from progression or overgrowth of a previous spinal fusion, or hyperthrophic osteophyte which may coexist with peridural scarring compressing significantly the dural elements[22]. Although bony and ligamentum compression may be mechanically reduced, pain relief may be minimal. This is one of the most difficult conditions to treat, whether conservatively or surgically, as the reduced diameter of the spinal canal makes any procedure (laminectomy, epidural injections, etc.) more difficult to perform and with greater chances for an incidental dural puncture[67]. In most instances the canal has a triangular shape instead of the usual round or oval morphology (Figure 26). Symptoms are magnified by this abnormal anatomy that makes the canal smaller than in normal individuals. Decompressive operations such as bilateral laminotomy may solve this problem temporarily, to the risk of rendering the vertebral segment instable and not uncommonly the eventual development of scarring and fibrosis which may eventually produce unilateral traction of the sac ensuing in symptoms of radiculopathy. Repeat intervention is likely to find abundant posterior fibrosis increasing the possibility of an incidental dural tear.

Pseudomeningocele

May occur after laminectomies[59,60] or fusions usually from unsealed dural tears followed by postural cephalea with or without CSF seeping through the incision[61,13]. If superficial layers are tightly closed CSF accumulates in the peridural region surrounding the pseudomeningocele[114,115] (Figure 9 and 10). Palpation of the area is very painful. Repair is difficult with high incidence of recurrence[113,116]. The size and location vary depending on the stage of development as they usually tend to decrease in size as time goes by, depending on the size of the connecting canal with the intradural subarachnoid space (Figure 27).

A variety of repair techniques have been proposed including a special clip, glues, drainage of the CSF for several days in attempts to stop the leak[118]. Occasionally one or two nerve rootlets are trapped within the sac, making surgical repair imperative as they need to be returned to the dural sac. Otherwise, spontaneous closure may eventually occur with only gently pressure applied with an elastic brace, for several weeks or months[119].

Surgery at the wrong level

Indeed the surgeon's nightmare can occur as sometimes the S1-S2 space is mobile or the L5-S1 space is non-mobile misleading the surgical team[4,22]. The only way to avoid operating in the wrong space is by confirming the precise location of the intervertebral space to be operated on. The best way is by placing a metal object (hemostat) in the intended space to be operated, then taking a radiograph or using a two-view fluoroscopy[66]. Errors are likely to occur when microdiskectomies are done, where exposure is marginal and fluoroscopy guidance depends on the interpretation of the operator[26].

Arachnoiditis

Is now been recognized as a serious complication of spinal operations since its existence has evolved from being questioned, ignored and overlooked to recognition as one of the most common complications. The permanent clinical syndrome has disastrous consequences on patients and enormous expense to the health care system, as it is not curable. A definite incidence has not been determined but isolated series have indicated that it occurs in 6 to 16% of the patients having lumbar laminectomies and in 11 to 29% of the patients that undergo spinal fusions[19,59,61]. One of the most revealing studies was conducted by Matsui et al[120] who obtained a lumbar spine MRI on the 3rd, 7th, 21st and 42nd day in 10 patients (7 for HNP and 3 for spinal stenosis) that sustained posterior approach spinal surgery. In axial views, intrathecal adhesions to the cauda equina were prevalent at the "laminectomized" levels in all patients. Partial adhesions were found at [9] levels, six weeks after surgery. Most of these resolved by the 42nd day, but in 5 out of 14 spaces exposed, partial nerve root adhesions were still present. An initial shrinking of the dural sac returned to near normal levels at the end of the observation period. This study showed that some of these changes are transitory; however, intradural lesions (clumped nerve roots) are evident even when only extradural surgery had been performed (Figure 14). The possible mechanisms for these events have been described in the section on intrathecal and extradural hematoma[62,68]; nevertheless, it is obvious that that the process is more complicated, involving wound bleeding[68], altered vascular permeability[121], inflammation[81] and the tissue injury cascade that follows[36,76,122].

Nakano et al[121] reported that laminectomy in rats, consistently induced an increase in vascular permeability in the cauda equina, as well as an increase in the vesicular transport of the endothelial cells with opening of the "tight junction", which suggests a breakdown of the blood-nerve barrier, facilitating the formation of adhesions. Furthermore, the same group[81] was able to show that the administration of the anti-inflammatory indomethacin and methylprednisolone, 24 hours after laminectomy, suppressed the formation of such adhesions and the leakage from the nutrient vessels. This phenomenon was only reduced when the drugs were given 3 or 6 weeks after laminectomy.

The importance of conducting serial neurological exams in patients that appeared to develop postoperative neurologic deficits[123] and to obtain imaging studies (preferably an MRI with contrast that may show enhanced nerve roots) of the operated region[78,124], is crucial in patients that may be suspected of having acute postoperative radicular irritation by the appearance of severe lumbar spine pain and neurologic deficits (Figure 30) after laminectomy, can not be overemphasized[125]. This premise also applies to cases of arachnoiditis in patients that had just received a fusion, with bone or titanium hardware. If the devices are made of other metals, a myelogram, followed by a CAT scan would be necessary in order to visualize the intrathecal structures. Early manifestations would be swollen, enhanced nerve roots that may be located in their normal position or in the anterior half of the sac[78,124,125] (Figure 30). Depending on the extent and intensity of the inflammatory reaction, clumping of nerve roots is not seen clearly until two or three months after the adverse event (Figure 31 and 32). Thereafter, the swelling gradually subsides and the nerve roots remain adhered to each other in clumps or to the interior wall of the dural sac 12°. This is a permanent condition. Although arachnoiditis is not present in every case of FBSS, nevertheless it complicates the clinical features of the latter making the differential diagnosis difficult, especially if metal hardware has been implanted. It also appears after exploration of the dural sac to remove hematomas, tumors, granulomas and other intrathecal lesions. At present, operations on the spine, seem to be the most common cause of cases of arachnoiditis

Distal dural sac ectasia

More often than not, the peridural fibrosis that follows any intervention on the spine, produces a certain degree of stenosis, impeding the normal circulatory return of the CSF converting the usual tapering of the dural sac into an ectasia of its caudal end expanding some times into a major dilatation (Figures 32 and 33). This complication has not been previously recognized as a pain generator manifesting itself as a severe pressure sensation (Figure 34) that exacerbates the low back pain[126]; pain on the lower extremities may or may not be present. Further operations, including fusions, will probably worsen this complication as the scarring most likely will increase. Re-operation to relieve the pain is futile unless this problem is relieved by derivation (lumbar-to-peritoneal shunt) of the retained CSF. Excision of the scar tissue by sharp dissection usually ends in another dural rent(s) and reappearance of scarring and fibrosis within four to six months.

Larger dilatations of the dural sac have been termed ectasia, having the same mechanism, but due to a greater degree of proximal constriction, it results in a larger distal dilatation of the sac (Figure 32). Other less common complications may be part of the FBSS, however because of their rarity they are not mentioned here.

Diagnosis

4

Practitioners need to have a precise understanding of this disease, as it usually includes a number of diagnosis that have been globalized in the "failed back surgery syndrome". Since adequate non-invasive procedures are available, to further subject these patients to invasive tests such as differential spinal or epidural blocks, discograms or neuroplasties will not only be futile and wasteful but they are hazardous as well[29,31,127].

A complete, detailed history obtained in chronological order, including diagnostic tests, adverse events, and attempted therapeutic modalities need to be listed, as well as, falls, minor injuries, work accidents, as trivial as they may appear, may give clues for the explanation of the actual patient's complaints. When fusions were followed by neurological deficit, it is important to find out if monitoring of spinal evoked potentials was done during the operative period[128,129,130]. Specific tracking of the time of appearance of symptoms in relation to one of the operations or any other spinal interventions performed may not only be a determinant of the cause of the FBSS, but may also assist in confirming or eliminating certain therapeutic modality that has not been of benefit in the past (Table 1). Repeated operations may produce both axial and radicular pain that may be caused from progression or overgrowth of a previous spinal fusion[51], or the presence of a hypertrophic osteophyte which may, in addition to peridural scarring, compress the dural contents[36,94]. Although compression from bone and hypertrophic ligaments may be mechanically reduced, pain relief would likely be nil[100].

After having one spinal operation, symptoms may be classified as:

- Mechanical, noted as increased back pain when standing or walking or sitting.
- Related, includes referred pain, muscle spasms, pain on the hips, or sacroiliac joints, or from bone friction as in pseudoarthrosis.
- Neurologic, including electrical shock-like, burning or lacerating pain, from stretching of the dural sac or the nerve roots and numbness or weakness not following a dermatome path.
- Radicular, including pain, sensory alteration (numbness, tingling, formication, etc) and weakness along a specific dermatome, usually due to extradural compression of a nerve root.
- Functional, implying dysfunction of bladder, bowel, sexual activities, autonomic dysfunction (excessive sweating, heat intolerance, hypertension).
- Aggregated, caused by other related illnesses like diabetic neuropathy, rheumatoid arthritis, osteoarthritis, lupus erythematosus, etc.
- Psychogenic, such as fears, depression, anxiety, hopelessness, insomnia, suicidal ideation and others.

Patients with recurrent low back pain after laminectomy that have several of these clinical manifestations require early consultation, prompt diagnosis, understanding and guidance. An algorythm to identify the possible cause of reappearing pain is shown in Table 1.

A detrimental trend has been the globalization of the radiological findings referred to by radiologists as "surgical changes", or "peridural enhancement, these statements are difficult to understand and to interpret for the average non-radiologist physician. There is an imperative need to have detailed and precise description of all the abnormal and out of the ordinary findings; furthermore a detailed description of any findings, level by intervertebral level, in the narrative manner, as well as a complete listing of the various diagnoses with opinions regarding their possible cause and without ignoring those age related changes. There is need to describe the location and extent of peridural fibrosis, to point out if there is distal dural sac dilatation (Figure 33) and to compare it (by actual measurement) with previous examinations to define if the width of the sac has increased in diameter, distal to where the surgery took place, as it is reflected by an annoying sensation of pressure in the lumbo-sacral area.

It is also important to recognize if the dural sac is adhered to one or both of the lamina, in which case, that level should be avoided in attempts to perform epidural injections and for surgeons planning to re-explore at that level. In axial views, the accurate description of the location (right, left or central) of clumped nerve roots, as well as their symmetry, or the lack of it. In sagittal views, the thickness and location of the nerve roots would also guide the clinicians as to where to or not to intervene. In essence, knowing those fine details might prevent the occurrence of incidental dural tears or punctures and complications that may result in further neurological injury. By the same token, it would be of value for radiologists to indicate at what levels are the widest posterior epidural spaces, so as to give the treating pain management physician guidance where is the dura, less likely to be punctured. Similarly, it would be useful to mention if there is a visible posterior epidural space, at the L5-S1 level and to indicate the distance from skin-to-epidural space.

In a retrospective review of the medical records of 684 patients, diagnosed with FBSS[131], after obtaining a history and performing a physical exam followed by imaging studies, the number and percentage of the possible pain generators was identified correlating them with location, extent and side of the clinical symptoms; revealed multiple pain generators in these patients (Table 2).

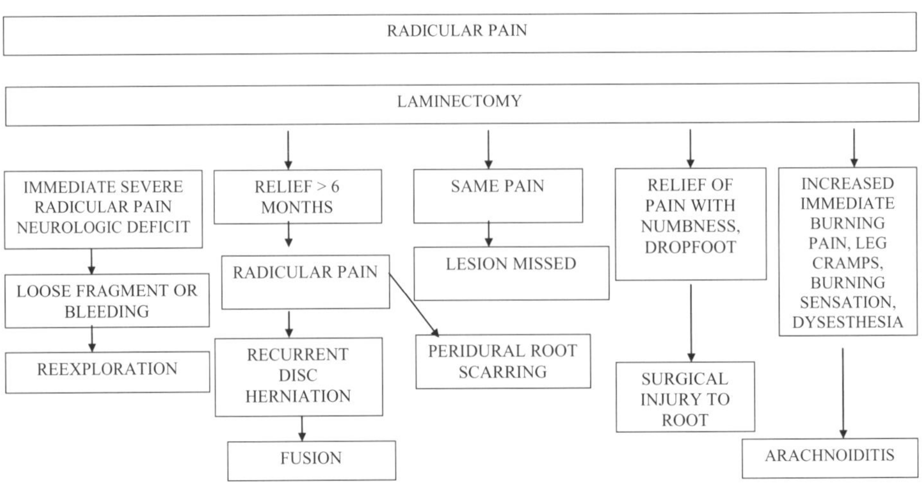

Table 1: Algorith for the diagnosis of postlaminectomy complications

From this data, there was no intention to establish incidence of post-laminectomy complications as the surgical interventions were performed by different surgeons and in different hospitals. Since some of these pain generators are not surgically correctable, patients with FBSS need to be informed that the presenting symptom, PAIN will likely continue after any subsequent operation. A list of specific diagnosis present is preferable, avoiding the generalized and imprecise diagnosis of FBSS.

Currently, since we have access to objective radiological findings as evidence of what the various diagnosis are, the so called "Waddell signs evaluation" may be deleted as it was based on non-organic, attitudinal and preconceived notions[132]. Although Waddell and Richardson[133] had already expressed certain doubt regarding the reliability of this questionable assessment of the symptoms and signs described and exhibited by the patient. Polatin et al[134], in their controlled, prospective study, performed in patients with low back pain, noted the lack of consistency by the evaluating physician. Currently, when we have precise means to establish accurate diagnosis, this guessing method is unacceptable.

Radiological findings	Number	Percentage
Epidural Scarring	578	84.5
Recurrent HNP	316	46.1
Dural Sac Ectasia	297	43.4
Deformity of Dural Sac	219	32.0
Herniation at adjacent Disk	194	28.3
Arachnoiditis	166	24.2
Spinal Instability	104	15.2
Facetectomy	78	11.4
Fusion with Hardware	64	9.3
Bony Fusion	32	4.6
Pseudomeningocele	21	3.0
Loose Disk Fragment	6	0.87

Table 2: Possible pain generators noted in imaging studies*

(*) Most patients had more than two pain generators[131]

Prognosis

5

The prediction herein expressed relates only to patients that have already been assigned the diagnosis of having failed back surgery syndrome. Unfortunately, the prognosis is not hopeful, at present time, since by definition, the label implies a hopeless condition, essentially condemning these patients to severe chronic pain, dysfunction and disability.

Attempts to identify the factors that predominantly affect the symptomatology seen in patients that undergo resection of the protruding portion of an intervertebral disk have shown that proportionally men usually have greater canal compromise than women[39,95] and a greater positive sciatic nerve tension[76,135]; both of which correlated with larger disk herniations. In non-operated groups, shorter duration of sciatica symptoms predicted good outcomes[136]. Moreover, younger patients with symptoms that lasted less than six months had better outcomes and no litigation. In contrast, larger discs, in relation to the vertebral canal diameter[6,137], cigarette smoking[35], involvement in litigation[3] and late middle age[6] were bad predicaments. For the operated groups, larger antero-posterior diameter and smaller central and paracentral herniations had better outcomes, while concurrent and pre-existent diseases, cigarette smoking, spondylosis, workers compensation claims, and middle age females had poorer outcomes[103,137]. These findings confirm that morphometric features of disk herniation, as they relate to the dimensions of the spinal canal, evident in MR imaging, appear to be the most reliable predictors [93,94].

The volume of complex operations performed by one specific surgeon, in one specific hospital have been shown to impact the outcomes of most operations[1,2,25]. It is now evident that patients with obesity, tobacco smoking, osteoporosis and certain congenital anatomical variances such as short vertebral pedicles, spondylosis, the presence of a rudimentary disk between S1-S2, lateral recess stenosis and mild scoliosis of the lumbar region have greater predisposition to post-laminectomy complications ending in FBSS[19,138]. In essence patients with one or more of these negative predictive factors ought to have surgical interventions in the spine, only after all conservative measures have been exhausted, as a last resource and with full understanding of the odds against their complete recovery.

Sadly as it is, we must accept that the precise etiology of some of the complications of lumbar spine surgery remain unresolved; the eventual outcomes, as they relate to pain relief, restoration of all functions and need for stronger opiate analgesics remain uncertain[107]. Solutions and answers to the following premises must be considered:

- Little advancement has been made in preventing or even reducing peridural fibrosis and scarring[26,32,33,62,122]
- The why and how some patients develop arachnoiditis after the most simple, apparently uncomplicated laminectomy are unanswered (see Figure 37)[120,121]

- Lack of definition as to whether "incidental dural tears" are likely to occur because of dural fragility or because of less than meticulous surgical technique[60,61]
- Why hardware, even when properly implanted appears to contribute to vertebral stress shielding, producing pain and loosening of even titanium screws, within two years post-implantation[139]
- Once installed, the hardware has been shown to serve as an on going, constant irritant to the overlying paraspinal muscles[122]
- No answer has been given to the postulate that pedicular screws, when placed closed to the lateral recess, block the venous channels within the pedicle leading to increased venous pressure, engorgement and altered blood flow resulting in localized pain[104,113]
- Evidence of corrosion and shielding of the metal used occurs in most cases, even when titanium is used[104,107,108].
- Since it has been shown that over 40% of screws are placed out of center, direct nerve injury is feasible[140,141]
- Pedicular microfractures occurring when the diameter of the screw is too large, in relation to the diameter of the pedicle, are difficult to recognize intraoperatively and nearly impossible to diagnose postoperatively[50,142,145]
- Posterior spinal instrumentation decreases the biomechanical properties of the ligamentum flavum, the posterior longitudinal ligament and the supraspinous ligament[43]
- Retrieval of the distal portion of a fracture's screw is difficult[139]
- Paravertebral muscle injury produced by desinsertion from bone and retraction pressure occurs in all patients that undergo posterior lumbar surgery and is aggravated by the number of spaces operated and the time of operation[122]
- Adjacent-disk-segment breakdown is more likely to occur in the immediately contiguous disk in 37% of patients that undergo spinal fusions (possibly from overuse)[90]
- Approximately 25% of patients that have spinal fusions will require another operation within one year[1,2,4,90,91]
- Lumbo-sacral spine fusions may indirectly cause stress-type fractures of the pelvic ring in elderly patients[143]
- In spite its proven efficacy in reducing inadvertent neurological injuries, during spinal fusions, SSEP monitoring has not been imposed as the standard of care[129,130]
- Cigarette smoking patients should be informed of the unfavorable prognosis they will have, unless they cease their habit, especially the high rate of fusions failure[35,41,42,43]
- Government agencies and insurers have not determined why is it that Americans need to have their spines operated eight fold more than populations in other industrialized countries[20,23]
- After having spine fusions, patients with pain-related symptoms should have, in addition to flexion-extension plain films, CAT Scans or MRI every four months for proper follow up

Treatment

6

Prevention is the best treatment, though a constellation of therapeutic modalities have been attempted in effort to relieve pain, the most significant manifestation of this disease. However, most of them have proven to be not only palliative, but also have been inadequately evaluated as the determination of evidence-based effectiveness[1,27,29,31]. In most cases therapeutic approaches have been less than satisfactory including intrathecal[144] or epidural infusions of opiates[145], spinal cord stimulation[146,147], sympathetic blocks[148], epidural injections of steroids[149] and anti-inflammatory drugs[150], phenol epidural injections[151] and others which provide only temporary relief of some of the patients' symptoms. A simplified guideline for the diagnostic and treatment of the most common cases is outlined in Table 3.

Presumptive diagnosis	Diagnostic tests	Initial therapy	Extended therapy
Retained Disk	H&P, MRI	Re-exploration	Analgesics, Anticonvulsants
Fragment or Foreign Body	CAT scan	Removal	Single Dose of Steroids IV
Periradicular Fibrosis	H&P, MRI	Analgesics, MgO_2 Epidural Steroids	Antiinflamatories, Muscle Relaxants, Anticonvulsants
Pseudomeningocele	H&P, MRI	Binder, Bed rest Decompression Anticonvulsants	Surgical Repair, Analgesics Bed rest, Anticonvulsants Acetazolamide
Nerve Root Cyst	H&P, MRI Myelogram	Analgesics, binder	Surgical Resection or Disk Plication
Spinal Stenosis	H&P, X- rays MRI or CAT Scan	Analgesics, MgO_2 Muscle Relaxants	Peridural Steroid Surgical Decompression
Arachnoiditis	H&P, MRI	Analgesics, MgO_2 Anticonvulsants IV Steroids x 5 days	Analgesics, Oral Steroids for flair ups, Anticonvulsants

Table 3: Guide to diagnosis and therapy of failed back syndrome

Lesions	Control measurement	Lumbar epidural	Caudal epidural	Transforaminal	Paravertebral
HNP + Radiculopathy	3.1 (±0.12)	7.2 (±0.51)	6.7 (±0.54)	7.4 (±0.9)	65.8 (±1.3)
FBS + Radiculopathy	2.9 (±0.09)	6.3 (±1.01)	5.8 (±0.3.4)	7.3 (±0.81)	6.1 (±0.72)

Table 4: Changes in pain progress score* in patients having injections of steroids through different approaches in patients with hnp vs those with fbs, all with lumbar radiculopathy**

**From J. A. Aldrete: The Pain Progress Score. A tool to measure therapeutic progress. Reg Anesth 1995:20:55.*
***Total score values obtained at evaluation, before and three weeks after each treatment.*

The possible benefit of lumbar epidural injections of steroids was studied in a comparative study in groups of patients with the diagnosis of FBSS versus herniated nucleus pulposus (HNP) that were treated by either epidural, caudal, transforaminal or paravertebral approaches, using the changes on the Pain Progress Score as a determinant of efficacy[152]. There were no significant differences in the benefit obtained from any of the techniques used as shown in the results presented in Table 4. Although, this outcome may be considered irrelevant, the importance of this study was that it showed, that regardless of the route of administration, the patients had the same degree of temporary improvement; however the likelihood of dural or nerve root puncture with paravertebral injections is nil, whereas with all the other approaches, either of these two complications, would aggravate the patient's condition.

The specific evaluating tool that we use as guide to determine either improvement or the lack of, with the therapeutic conduct to follow is the Pain Progress Score that utilized five parameters, each of which contained three different components to which values 0, 1 or 2 are assigned[152]. The sum of the five parameters indicates the total condition of the patient and by comparing it with the total scores of previous treatments, it is possible to define if the patient is improving or getting worse, and specifically in which particular aspect of the evaluation is the patient affected. (Table 5)

		1st visit	2nd visit	3rd visit	4th visit	5th visit
Pain intensity	**(0) 8 to 10 level (1) 5 to 7 level (2) 0 to 3 level**					
Physical activity	**(0) Activities severely limited by pain (1) Activities slightly limited by pain s (2) Able to perform all expected activities**					
Emotional attitude	**(0) Severely depressed (1) Mild depression (2) Adapts well and copes with pain**					
Analgesic intake	**(0) Parenteral opiod (1) Oral opioid analgesic (2) NSAID or nonopioid analgesic**					
Other pain-related medications	**(0) Tranquilizers, hypnotics, muscle relaxants, anti-depressants, others (1) Muscle relaxants, anti-depressants (2) Muscle relaxants only**					
Total score						

Table 5: The pain progres score. Aldrete pain progress score ©. *From Aldrete JA. The pain progress score: a tool to measure therapeutic progress. Regional anesthesia, 20 (S2): 55, 1995.*

Many other attempts to relief the pain in patients with FBSS have proven limited in duration and scope; on this matter, it remains an essential guide the main premise of the Hypocratic Oath: *prima non-nocere*; in other words, because we are trying to relieve these patients pain, we are not justified to undertake risky procedures or even certain procedures that although, rarely may cause worse injury to these patients, but frequently have little benefit (i.e. neuroplasty[153,154], discography[155], epidural steroid injections[156], etc.). Whatever if it is to be attempted, it must have been proven that it will result in an obvious benefit, without risk.

Other forms of therapy using neurolytic substances[151,157,158] have a high risk of injury with a low benefit ratio. Further surgical interventions are only indicated when absolutely necessary, such as in the case of a loose disk fragment compressing a nerve root, sudden sensory or motor deficit, loss of sphincter control, large epidural abscess or hematomas that because of potential irreversible neural damage, may require immediate surgical intervention.

When fusions include implanted hardware, a screw may be pressing on a nerve root if mal-positioned (Figure 1) or if there is a screw fracture, removal may also be indicated. Since fusions have not been proven to be cost effective, have a high incidence of complications, require more subsequent surgical interventions and specifically because of failure to relieve the patient's chief complaint, pain, Deyo et al[1,2] have emphasized that research should be on why and who should undergo fusion, rather than how to perform another fusion. Destructive or neuroablative procedures are not recommended as they may result in added morbidity and neural deficit[157,158].

The accurate selection of patient candidates for spinal surgery is crucial to prevent further increases in the population of patients with FBSS; the aims of the operative procedure need to be reevaluated, focusing on the elimination of pain rather than on the technical success of the operation. Implantation of hardware and spinal interventionism have to be proven with randomized and not randomized controlled trials, including at least 400 patients in each group, with a follow up of at least two years, in the hope that the results provide obvious scientific evidence that they are efficacious in relieving pain and improving the physical condition of the patient[159,160] and not ending in the subgroup of patients "thrown in the pool" of failed back surgery syndrome, before publicizing and generalizing their application[161,162,163,164,165].

Lack of in-depth interpretation of radiological films whether plain roentgenograms, MRI or CAT scans, place the treating physicians at a disadvantage and the patients in jeopardy. Still not addressed in Deyo et al's review[1] are the incidence of neurological deficits, vascular injuries, arachnoiditis, epidural and extradural hematomas; hardware breakage, slippage, migration, biomechanical failure, malpositioning, removal before two years, nor CSF leakage, pseudomeningocele, infections (Figure 36), pseudoarthrosis, bladder, bowel and sexual dysfunction, etc.

The metallic hardware makes subsequent, identification of intrathecal structures difficult; myelography followed by CAT scan and MRI still show considerable distortion of images, making precise diagnosis not feasible, leaving patients with frank radicular symptoms in a quandary.

The prespective and the obligation of having to treat these patients for long periods of time, is different from the enthusiastic reports by those who implanted them. To obtain appropriate data, they should also be followed by an impartial and objective group, for periods longer than two years. The burden of proof, whether patients are improved by these procedures or not, should fall on the surgeons who perform and advocate these procedures. Clinical success was only 57% in patients that have had surgery before, which is most of the cases[166].

There is need for a National Spine Fusion Registry that impartially and objectively will verify the improvement of these patients, every six months, for at least three years after surgery, keeping track of the type of instrumentation done, the complications that develop and the type of re-operations that were needed. The indications for lumbar fusion with hardware need to be re-evaluated, considering that as long as the patient's pain persists, whatever procedure performed failed. Most studies published, about spinal fusions of the lumbar spine, with hardware, are flawed because they lack:

a) Consistent selection of patients
b) Minimal audit of the participating surgeons
c) No independent evaluation of radiographs, nor of patients outcome
d) Include fewer than 400 patients.
e) Inadequate statistically significance analysis was conducted in most of the studies
f) There was no randomization
g) Radiological confirmation of complications is difficult because of metal hardware
h) Plain films were frequently not interpreted by a radiologist
i) The majority of studies do not have the characteristics required to be part of meta-analysis

Once more, in their long list of contributions analyzing the subject of low back pain, Deyo and cols[1] have made a valiant, comprehensive and objective review of the ever growing and questionable indications for and the results from spinal fusions. They pointed out the lack of properly conducted studies typical of this aspect of spinal surgery, as most of the studies showed considerable number of patients "lost", with the remainder of the subjects had questionable outcomes since low back pain was not included in the evaluation criteria[5,49,50,52,167], nevertheless, the results in the remaining patients were labeled as "satisfactory".

7 Conclusions

The broadly unspecific diagnosis of "failed back syndrome" is perhaps partly responsible for the diversity of results obtained from most of the therapeutic modalities that have been recommended to treat it. It is crucial that a precise diagnosis is made including all possible pain generators and originators of disability attempting to identify their location and the extent of the lesion(s), plus added pathology such as S-I joint degeneration, spondylosis, spondylolisthesis, spinal stenosis, etc.

Since diagnostic procedures have multiplied, it is our obligation to choose the one that would afford the most information for a reasonable cost, with the least risk. Provocative procedures render little information and have the doubt of having being done by the same individual that will interpret them and will proceed to perform what ever definite operation will follow. The possible congenital variances, present in about 30% of the general population tend to affect laminectomies outcome because they produce instability of the segment and result in an accelerated degeneration of the disk just above the operated level which will undoubtedly affect each patient's recovery. To reduce the unknown incidence of FBSS, the unfavorable prognostic factors present in each patient will have to be identified before surgical intervention, as they would greatly influence the eventual outcome of the first and every operation, from then on.

Transient fads such as electrical stimulation to accelerate bone growth in fusions proved to be useless, prolonged surgery time and increased the cost of the intervention[84,164,165]. New plates and screws[166] or interbody replacement discs[48,50,55,102] have to be evaluated objectively. Undue injuries during surgery could be prevented by the routine use of dermatomal evoked responses, specifically during the insertion of transpedicular screws in the lumbosacral spine. This precaution should be established as the standard of care to avoid nerve root injury.

Much needs to be learned from proper studies conducted on chronic, severe low back pain that will include systematic reviews of randomized control trials and meta-analyses of groups and subgroups having identifiable pathological process. It is obvious that precise and unquestionable diagnosis ought to precede any therapy that otherwise would be blinded and without a definite target; then we will be practicing evidence-based medicine.

References

1. Deyo RA, Nachefson A, Mirza SK. Spinal fusion surgery - the case for restraint. N Eng J Med 2004: 350: 722-726.
2. Deyo RA, Ciol MA, Cherkin DC, et al. Lumbar spinal fusion: a cohort study of complications, re-operation and resource use in the Medicare population. Spine 1993:18:1463-1470.
3. Leboeuf-Yde C, Kyvik KO. When does low back pain become a common problem? A study of 29,424 individuals aged 12-41 years. Spine 1998: 23: 228-34.
4. Wilkinson HA. The failed back syndrome. Springer-Verlag, New York. 1983: pp. 2-15.
5. North RB, Campbell JN, Javers CS et al. Failed back surgery síndrome: a 5-year follow-up in 102 patients undergoing repeated operations. Neurosurgery 1991: 28: 685-691.
6. Taylor VM, Deyo RA, Ciol M, et al. Patient-oriented outcomes from low back surgery. Spine 2000: 25: 19: 2445-2452.
7. Deyo RA, Weinstein JN. Low back pain. N Eng J Med 2001:344:363-70.
8. Ostello RW, de Vet HC, Waddell G, et al. Rehabilitation following first-time lumbar disk surgery: a systematic review within the frame work of the Cochrane collaboration. Spine 2003: 28: 209-18.
9. Quinke H. Ueber Lumbalpunction. Berlin Klin Wochen 1891: 28: 889-891.
10. Dandy WE: Roentgenography of the brain after the injection of air into the spinal canal. Ann Surg 1919; 70: 397-403.
11. Sicard JA, Forestier J. Methode general d'exploration radiologique parl'huide iodee (Lipiodol) Bull Med Soc Hop Paris 1922: 46: 463-469.
12. Dale AJ, Love JG. Thorium dioxide myelopathy. JAMA 1967:199:606-60
13. Aldrete JA. Myelography. In Arachnoiditis: the silent epidemic. Aldrete JA (ed), Futuremed, Denver. 2000: pp. 41-63.
14. Mixter WJ, Barr JS. Rupture of the intervertebral disk with involvement of the spinal canal. N Eng J Med 1934: 211:210-214.
15. Ramsey GH, French JD, Strain WH. Iodinated organic compounds as contrast media for radiographic diagnosis. IV Pantopaque myelography. Radiology 1944: 43: 236-240.
16. Luce JC, Leith W, Burrage WS. Pantopaque meningitis due to hypersensitivity. Radiology 1951: 57: 879-871.
17. Imielinski L, Chmielewski JM. Arachnoidite adhesive intraarachidienne a la suite de myelographies a l' ethiodane (Pantopaque). J Radiol Electrol Med Nucl 1971: 52: 31-43.
18. Quiles M, Marchisello PJ, Tsairis P. Lumbar adhesive arachnoiditis: Etiologic and pathologic aspects. Spine 1978: 3:45-50.

19. Zeidman SM, Long DM. Failed back surgery syndrome. In: Menezes AHJ, Sonntag VKH, (eds) Principles of Spinal Surgery. New York, McGraw-Hill. 1996: 657-80.
20. Franklin GM, Haug JA, Heyer NJ, McKeefrey S, Picciano JF. Outcome of lumbar fusion in Washington State Workers' Compensation. Spine 1994:19:1897-904, 1903. VKH, eds. Principles of Spinal Surgery. New York: McGraw-Hill, 1996: 657-680.
21. Carrol SE, Wiesel SW. Neurological complications and lumbar laminectomies. Clin Orthop 1992: 25: 14-23.
22. Long D. Failed back surgery syndrome. Neurosurg Clin N Am 1991: 2: 899-903.
23. Cherkin DC, Deyo RA, Loeser JD, et al. An international comparison of back surgery rates. Spine 1994: 19: 1201-6.
24. Dugan SA, Frost DA, Sullivan KP. An active and cost-conserving approach to the management of low back pain. Hospital Physician 2002: 55-66.
25. Volinn E. The epidemiology of low back pain in the rest of the world. Spine 1997: 22: 1747-1754.
26. Wilkinson HA. The role of improper surgery in the etiology of the failed back syndrome. In The Failed Back Syndrome, Wilkinson HA (ed); 2nd edition. Springer-Verlag, New York. 1992: pp. 4-12.
27. Turner JA, Loeser JD, Bell KG. Spinal cord stimulation for chronic low back pain: a systematic literature syntesis. Neurosurgery 1995: 37: 1088-95.
28. Merril DG. Hoffman's glasses: Evidence-based medicine and the search for quality in the literature of Intervencional Pain Medicine. Reg Anesth Pain Med, 2003: 28: 547-60.
29. Turk DC. Clinical effectiveness and cost effectiveness of treatments of patients with chronic pain. Clin J Pain 2002: 18: 355-65.
30. Steffee AD, Biscup RS, Sitowski DJ. Segmental spine plates with pedicular screw fixation. A new internal fixation device for disorders of the lumbar and thoracolumbar spine. Clin Ortho Rel Res 1986: 203: 45-51.
31. Cherkin DC, Deyo RA, Battie ML, et al. A comparison of physical therapy, chiropractic manipulation, and provision of an educational booklet for the treatment of patients with low back pain. N Eng J Med 1998: 339: 1021-9.
32. Matsui H, Kanamori M, Kawaguchi Y, et al. Clinical and electrophysiologic characteristics of compressed lumbar nerve roots. Spine 1997: 22: 2100-2105.
33. Hardy RW. Extradural cauda equina and nerve root compression from benign lesions of the lumbar spine. In Neurological Surgery, Youmans JR (ed), 4th ed.; W. B. Saunders, Co., Philadelphia. 1996: pp. 2368-2372.
34. Albin MS, Bunegain L, Marlin A, et al. Brain retraction pressure and cerebral perfusion. Anesthesiology 1980: 53: S117.
35. Bom CW, Orme TJ, Richardson D. The rate of pseudoarthrosis in patients who are smokers and in patients that are not smokers. A comparison study. Spine 1986: 11: 11: 942-3.
36. Wilkinson HA. Diagnostic Errors and Inadequate Surgery. In The failed back syndrome, 2nd ed. Wilkinson HA (ed) Springer Verlag, New York. 1992: pp. 26-31.
37. Whiteland TS, Butler JC, Cohen JL, et al. Complications with the variable spinal plating system. Spine 1989: 14: 472-476.
38. Cherkin DC, Deyo RA, Wheeler K, et al. Physician variation in diagnostic testing for low back pain: who you see is what you get. Arthritis Rheum 1994: 37: 15-22.

39. Carrage EJ, Chen Y, Tanner CA, et al. Provocative discography in patients after limited lumbar discography in patients after limited lumbar discectomy: A controlled randomized study of pain response in symptomatic and asymptomatic subjects. Spine 2000: 3065-71.
40. Woodside JR Jr. Females smokers have increase perioperative narcotic requirement. J Adict Dis 2000: 19: 1-10.
41. Silvertein P. Smoking and wound healing. Am J Med 1992: 93: 225-248.
42. Warner DO, Patten CA, Ames SC, et al. Smoking behaviour and perceived stress in cigarette smokers undergoing elective surgery. Anesthesiology 2004: 100: 1125-1137.
43. Silcox DH, Boden SD, Schimandle JH, et al. Osteoinductive protein extract. Spine 1998: 23: 291-7.
44. Kwaiatkowski TC, Hanley EN. Cigarette smoking and its orthopedic consequences. Am J Orthop 1996: 25: 590-597.
45. Pedicle Screws: FDA Medical Bulletin, 10 May, 1994.
46. Pohler OEM. Unalloyed titanium for implants in bone surgery. Injury 2000: 31: 7-13.
47. Hutton DC, Ganey TM, Elmer WA, et al. Does long-term compressive loading on the intervertebral disk cause degeneration. Spine 2000: 25: 2993-3004.
48. Geisler FH. Lumbar Artificial Disk Replacement with the Charité Artificial Disk. Advanced Medicine Journal, Summer 2005: 12-14.
49. Hinckley BS, Jaremko ME. Effects of 360-degree lumbar fusion in a worker's compensation population. Spine 1995: 20 Suppl 24: 1388-1428.
50. Cunningham BW, Sefter JC, Shono Y, McAfee PC. Static and Cyclical Biomechanical Analysis of Pedicle Screw Spinal Constructs. Spine 1993: 18: 12: 1677-1688.
51. Kestler OC. Overgrowth (hypertrophy) of lumbosacral grafts causing a complete spinal block. Bull Hosp Joint Dis 1966: 27: 51-57.
52. Benzel E, Sonntag VK, McCormcik P. A novel surgical treatment of lumbar disk herniation in patients with long-standing degenerative disk disease. Editorial J Neurosurg: Spine 2005: 2: 513-514.
53. Schneider EC, Zaslavsky AM, Epstein AM. Use of High-Cost Operative Procedures by Medicare Beneficiaries Enrolled in For-Profit and Not-for-Profit Healthe Plans. N Engl J Med 2004: 350: 2: 143-150.
54. Cunningham BW, Gordon JD, Dimitriev AE, et al. Biomechanical evaluation of total disk replacement arthroplasty: An in vitro human cadaveric model. Spine 2003: 28: 20S: S110-S117.
55. Kleuver M, Oner FC, Jacobs WC. Total disk replacement for low back pain: background and a systematic review of the literature. Eur Spine J 2003: 12: 108-116.
56. Deyo RA. Practice variations, treatment fads, raising disability. Do we need a new clinical research paradigm. Spine 1993: 18: 2153-62.
57. Van Tulder MW, Boes BW, Bouter LM. Conservative treatment of acute and chronic nonspecific low back pain: a systematic review of randomized control trials of the most common interventions. Spine 1997: 22: 2128-2156.
58. Eismont FJ, Wiesel SW, Rothman RH. Treatment of dural tears associated with spinal surgery. J Bone Joint Surg 1981: 63A: 1132-1136.
59. Jones AM, Stambough JL, Balderstyon RA, et al. Long-term results of lumbar spine surgery complicated by incidental durotomy. Spine 1989: 14: 443-446.

60. Goodkin R, Laska LL. Unintended "incidental" durotomy during surgery of the lumbar spine: medico-legal implications. Surg Neurol 1995: 43: 4-14.
61. Aldrete JA, Ghaly RF. Post-laminectomy pseudomeningocele: an unsuspected cause of low back pain. Reg Anesth 1995: 20:75-79.
62. La Rocca H, McNab I. The "laminectomy membrane" studies on its evolution, characteristics, effects and prophylaxis in dogs. J Bone Joint Surg 1974: 56: 545-550.
63. Hogland J, Freemont AJ, Denton J, et al. Retained surgical swab debris in post laminectomy arachnoiditis and peridural fibrosis. J Bone Joint Surg Br 1988: 70: 659-662.
64. Liu S, Boutrand JP, Bittoun J, Tadie M. A collage-based sealant to prevent in vivo reformation of epidural scar adhesions in an adult rat laminectomy model. J Neurosurg 2002: 97: 69-73.
65. Gawande AA, Studdert DM, Orav EJ, et al. Risk factors for retained instruments and sponges after surgery. N Eng J med 2003: 348: 229-235.
66. Schellinger D, Manz HJ, Vidic B, et al. Disk fragment migration. Radiology 1990: 175: 831-836.
67. Carrage EJ, Kim DH. A prospective analysis of MRI findings in patients with sciatica and lumbar disk herniation: Correlation of outcomes with disk fragment and canal morphology. Spine 1997: 22: 1650-1660.
68. DeLeo JA, Colburn RW. The role of cytokines in nociception and chronic pain. In Low Back Pain: A Scientific and Clinical Overview. Weinstein JN & Gordon SL. Am Acad Orthop Surg 1996: 163-185.
69. Borgeson SE, Vang PS. Extradural pseudocysts. Acta Orthop Scand 1973: 44: 12-20.
70. Yamagami T, Matsui H, Tsuji J, et al. Effects of laminectomy and retained extradural foreign body on cauda equina adhesion. Spine 1993: 18: 1774-1781.
71. Friedman J, Whitecloud TS III. Lumbar cauda equina syndrome associated with the use of gelfoam: case report. Spine 2001: 26: 485-487.
72. Kemaloglu S, Ozkan U, Yilmaz F, et al. Prevention of spinal epidural fibrosis by recombinant tissue plasminogen activator in rats. Spinal Cord 2003: 41: 430-431.
73. Oswald AM, Joly LM, Gurry C, et al. Fatal intraoperative anaphylaxis related to aprotinin after local application of fibrin glue. Anesthesiology 2003: 99: 521-523.
74. Brotchi JC, Pirotte B, DeWitt O, et al. Prevention of epidural fibrosis in prospective series of 100 primary lumbosacral discectomy patients: follow-up an assessment at reoperation. Neurol Res 1999: 21: 47-50.
75. Ghaly RF, Aldrete JA. Surgical treatment. In Arachnoiditis: the silent epidemic. Aldrete JA (ed) Futuremed, Denver, 2000: pp. 305-322.
76. Spencer DL, Irwin GS, Miller JA. Anatomy and significance of fixation of lumbosacral nerve roots in sciatica. Spine 1983: 8: 672-679.
77. Ross JS Masaryk TJ, Schrader M, et al. Imaging of the postoperative lumbar spine: assessment with gadopentetate dimeglumine. AJNR 1990: 11771-776.
78. Aldrete JA, Brown TL. Laboratory and radiological diagnosis. In Arachnoiditis: the silent epidemic. Aldrete JA (ed), Futuremed, Denver, 2000: 221-53.
79. Ross JS, Masaryk TJ, Modic MT, et al. MR imaging of lumbar arachnoiditis. AJR 1987: 149: 1025-1032.
80. Wilmink JT, Hofman PA. MRI of the postoperative lumbar spine: triple dose gadodiamide and fat suppression. Neuroradilogy 1997: 39: 589-592.

81. Nakano M, Matsui H, Miaki K, Tsuji H. Postlaminectomy adhesion of the cauda equina. Inhibitory effects of anti-inflammatory drugs on cauda equina adhesions in rats. Spine 1998: 23: 298-304.
82. Tarlov EC. Foraminal and extraforaminal lumbar disk herniation. Techniques in Neurosurgery. 1996: 2: 244-8.
83. Hardy RW. Far lateral disk herniation: illustrative cases. Techniques in Neurosurgery 1996: 2: 210-1.
84. McCormick PC. Lumbar stenosis decompression with fusion (no instrumentation). Techniques in Neurosurgery 1996: 2: 223-7.
85. Aldrete JA. Pain generators in failed back syndrome. Presented at the World Congress of the WFSA, Paris, France. April 21-25, 2004.
86. Kotani Y, Cunningham BW, Cappuccino A, et al. The effects of spinal fixation and destabilization on the biomechanical and histologic properties of spinal support. Spine 1998: 23: 672-83.
87. Roberts N, Gratin C, Whitehouse GH, et al. MRI analysis of lumbar intervertebral disk height in young and older populations. J Magnetic Res Imaging, 1997: 7: 880-886.
88. Panjabi MM, Oxland T, Yamamoto, et al. Mechanical behavior or the human lumbar spine and lumbosacral spine as shown by three-dimensional load displacement curves. J Bone Joint Surg 1994: 76: 413-424.
89. Fujiwara A, Lim T, An HS, et al. The effect of disk degeneration and facet joint osteoarthritis on the segmental flexibility of the lumbar spine. Spine: 2000: 23: 3036-3034.
90. Schlegel JD, Smith JA, Schleusener RL. Lumbar motion segment pathology adjacent to thoracolumbar, lumbar and lumbosacral fusions. Spine 1996: 21: 970-81.
91. Simeone F. Lumbar disk disease. In Neurosurgery, Wilkins RH and Rengachary SS (eds), 2nd ed. Vol. III. McGraw-Hill, New York. 1996: pp. 3805-3814.
92. Luoma K, Vehmas T, Raininko R, et al. Lumbosacral transitional vertebre: relation to disk degeneration and low back pain. Spine 2004: 29: 200-5.
93. Hinkley BS, Jarenko ME. The effects of 360-degree lumbar fusion in a worker's compensation population. Spine 1995: 24: Suppl. 128-142.
94. Ohnmeiss DD, Vanharata H, Ekholm J. Degree of disk disruption and lower extremity pain. Spine 1997: 22: 1600-1605.
95. Junge A, Dvorak J, Ahrens S. Predictors of bad and good outcomes of lumbar disk surgery. Spine 1995: 20: 460-486.
96. Bennett GJ, Serhan HA, Sorini PM, Willis BH. An experimental study of lumbar destabilization: Restabilization and bone density. Spine 1997: 22: 1448-1453.
97. Katler A, Wilke HJ, Dietl R, et al. Stabilizing effect of posterior lumbar interbody fusion cages before and after cyclic loading. J Neurosurg (Spine) 2000: 92: 87-92.
98. Heithoff KB, Burton CV. CT evaluation of the failed back surgery syndrome. Orth Clinics N Am 1985: 16: 417-44.
99. Rudish A, Kremser C, Peer S, Kathrein A. Imaging of patients with spinal fusion. Spine 1998: 12: 692-9.
100. Fritzell P, Hagg O, Nordwall A. Complications in lumbar fusion surgery for chronic low back pain: comparison of three surgical techniques used in a prospective randomized study. Eur Spine J 2003: 12: 178-189.
101. Henstorf JE, Gaines RW, Steffee AD. Transpedicular fixation of spinal disorders with Steffee plates. Surgical Rounds for Orthopaedics, March 1987.

102. Cunningham BW, Dmitriev AE, Hu N, McAfee PC. General principles of total disk replacement arthroplasty. Spine 2003: 28: 20S: S118-S124.
103. Edwards CC, Weigel MC. A prospective study of 51 low lumbar nonunions. Ortop Trans 1988: 12: 608-12.
104. Hallab NJ, Cunningham BW, Jacobs JJ. Spinal Implant Debris-Induced Osteolysis. Spine 2003: 28: 20: S125-S138.
105. Delamarter RB, Fribourgh DM, Kanim LEA, Bae H. ProDisc Artificial Total Lumbar Disk Replacement: Introduction and Early Results From the United States Clinical Trial. Spine 2003: 28:20:S167-S175.
106. Vlessides M. Practice-changing studies must be held to a higher standard. Anesthesiology News, January 2002: 11-12.
107. Thomsen K, Christensen FB, Eiskjaer SP, Hansen ES, Fruensgaard S, Bünger CE. 1997 Volvo Award Winner in Clinical Studies. The effect of pedicle screw instrumentation on functional outcome and fusion rates in posterolateral lumbar spinal fusion: a prospective randomized clinical study. Spine 1997: 22: 24: 2813-2821.
108. Mott JC, Wolfe SM. Investigation of pedicular (spinal) screw implantation. Public Citizens Dec. 20, 1994.
109. Martin RJ, Yuan HA. Neurosurgical care of spinal epidural, subdural and intramedullary abscesses and arachnoiditis. Orthop Clinic Nort Am 1993: 27: 125-136.
110. Linholm TS, Pylkkanen P. Discitis following removal of intervertebral disk. Spine 1982: 7: 617-682.
111. Maiuri F, Iaconetta G, Gallichio B, et al. Spondylodiscitis: clinical and MRI diagnosis. Spine 1997: 22: 1741-1746.
112. Aldrete JA, Williams SK. Infections from extended epidural catheterization in ambulatory patients. Reg Anesth Pain Med 1998: 23: 491-495.
113. Lee KS, Hardy IM II. Postlaminectomy lumbar pseudomeningocele: report of four cases. Neurosurgery 1992: 30: 111-4.
114. Nash CL, Kaufman B, Frankel VH. Postsurgical, meningeal pseudocyst of the lumbar spine. Surg Neurol 1971: 75: 167-78.
115. Hadami FG, Knoler N, Tadmor R, et al. Entrapped nerve root in pseudomeningocele after laminectomy. Report of three cases. Neurosurgery 1986: 19: 405-7.
116. Robertson JT, Soble-Smith J, Powsers N. Prevention of cerebrospinal fistulae and reduction of epidural scar with new surgical hemostat device in a porcine laminectomy model. Spine 2003: 28: 2298-303.
117. Prigor JJ, Wallace DJ, Harner A, et al. A sprayable hemostat containing fibrillar collagen. Ann Thor Surg 1999: 68: 479-85.
118. Kumar AJS, Nambiar CS, Kanse P. Spontaneous resolution of lumbar pseudomeningocele. Spinal Cord 2003: 41: 470-2.
119. Ivar Brox J, Sorenson R, Fris A, et al. Randomized clinical trial of lumbar instrumented fusion and cognitive intervention and exercises in patients with chronic low back pain and disk degeneration. Spine 2003: 28: 1913-1921.
120. Matsui H, Tsuji H, Kanamori M, et al. Laminectomy induced arachnoradiculitis: a postoperative serial MRI study. Neuroradiology 1995: 37: 660-666.
121. Nakano M, Matsui H, Miaki K, et al. Postlaminectomy adhesion of the cauda equina. Changes of postoperative vascular permeability of the cauda equina in rats. Spine 1997: 15: 22: 1005-1114.
122. Kawaguchi Y, Matsui H, Tsuji H. Back muscle injury after posterior lumbar spine surgery. Spine 1996: 21 941-4.

123. Garkin SR. Editorial. Spine 1994: 19: 2254-S.
124. Avidan A, Gomori M, Davison E. Nerve root inflammation demonstrated by MRI in a patient with transient neurologic symptoms after intrathecal injection of lidocaine. Anesthesiology 2002: 97: 257-258.
125. Aldrete JA. Nerve root "irritation" or inflammation diagnosed by MRI. Anesthesiology 2003: 98: 1294.
126. Aldrete JA. Severe lumbosacral spine pressure produced by postlaminectomy and or fusion distal sac dilatation. In Press.
127. Jadad AR, Browman GP. The WHO analgesic ladder for pain management. Stepping up the quality of its evaluation. JAMA 1995: 274: 1870-3.
128. Straham C, Min K, Boos N, et al. Reliability of perioperative SSEP recordings in spine surgery. Spinal Cord 2003: 41: 483-489.
129. Calencie B, Madsen P, Lebwohl N. Stimulus evoked EMG monitoring during transpedicular lumbosacral spine instrumentation. Clinical results. Spine 1994: 19: 2780-6.
130. Toleikis JR, Carlvin AO, Shapiro DE, et al. The use of dermatomal evoked responses during surgical procedures that use intrapedicular fixation of the lumbosacral spine. Spine 1993: 16: 24021-7.
131. Aldrete JA, Aldrete VT. Pain generators in patients with failed back syndrome. XIII Congress WFSA Paris, France April 22 to 27, 2004.
132. Waddell G, Mcculloch J, Kummel E, Venner R. Non-organic physical signs in low back pain. Spine. 1980: 5: 117-125.
133. Waddell G, Richardson J. Observation of overt pain behavior by physicians during routine clinical examination of patients with low back pain. J Psychosom Res 1992: 36: 77-87.
134. Polatin PB, Cox B, Gatchel RJ, Mayer TG. A Prospective study of Waddell signs in patients with chronic low back pain. Spine 1997: 22: 1618-1621.
135. Taylor VM, Deyo RA, Ciol M, et al. Patient-oriented outcomes from low back surgery: A community based study. Spine 2000: 23: 2445-52.
136. Jamner ID, Girdler SS, Shapiro D, Jarvik MI. Pain inhibition, nicotine and gender. Exp Clin Psychopharmacol 1998: 6: 96-106.
137. Porter R, Bewley B. A ten-year prospective study of vertebral canal size as a predictor of back pain. Spine 1994: 19: 173-175.
138. Carragene EJ. Persistent low back pain. N Eng J Med 2005: 352: 1891-8.
139. Di Lorenzo N, Conti R, Romoli S. Retrieval of broken pedicle screws by "friction techniques". J Neurosurg (Spine) 2000: 92: 114-6.
140. Kwok AWL, Finkelstein JA, Woodside T, Hearn TC, Hu RW. Insertional Torque and Pull-out Strengths of Conical and Cylindrical Pedicle Screws in Cadaveric Bone. Spine 1996: 21: 21: 2429-2434.
141. Castro HM, Halm A, Jerosch J, Malms J, Steinbeck J, Plasius S. Accuracy of pedicle screw placement in lumbar vertebrae.
142. Dick JC, Zdeblick TA, Bartel BD, Kunz DN. Mechanical evaluation of cross-link designs in rigid pedicle screw systems. Spine 1997: 22: 4: 370-375.
143. Wood KB, Geissele AE, Ogilvie JW. Pelvic fractures after long lumbosacral spine fusions. Spine 1996: 21: 1357-62.
144. Krames ES, Lanning RM. Intrathecal infusion of analgesics for non-malignant pain: Analgesic efficacy. J Pain Symptom Manage 1996: 8: 539-348.
145. Aldrete JA. Temporary epidural infusions in ambulatory patients with severe lumbalgia. Pain Reviews 1996: 3: 1-3.

146. Carter ML. Spinal cord stimulation in chronic pain: a review of the evidence. Anaesth Intensiv Care 2004: 32: 11-21.
147. Cameron T. Safety and efficacy of spinal cord stimulation for the treatment of chronic pain: a 20-year literature review. J Neurosurg (Spine) 2004: 254-263.
148. Fredman B, Zophar E, Nun MB, et al. The effect of repeated epidural sympathetic nerve block on "failed back surgery syndrome" associated with chronic low back pain. J Clin Anesth 1999: 11: 46-51.
149. Cluff R, Meshio AK, Cohen SP, et al. The technical aspects of epidural steroid injections: a national survey. Anesth Analg 2002: 95: 403-8.
150. Aldrete JA. Epidural injections of indomethacin for postlaminectomy syndrome: A preliminary report. Anesth Analg 2003: 96: 463-468.
151. Racz GB, Heavner JE, Haynsworth R. Repeat epidural phenol injection in chronic pain and spasticity. In techniques of neurolysis. Racz GB (ed.) Kluer Academic 1989: pp. 193-212.
152. Aldrete JA. Pain Progress Score: A tool to measure therapeutic progress. Reg Anesth 1995: 18: 55.
153. Heavner J, Racz GB, Singleton W, et al. Percutaneous epidural neuroplasty. Reg Anesth Pain med 1999: 24: 201-207.
154. Devulder J, Bogaet L, Castille F, et al. Relevance of epidurography and epidural adhesiolysis in chronic failed back surgery patients. Clin J Pain 1995: 11: 147-150.
155. Carragge EJ, Chen Y, Tanner CM, et al. Provocative discography in patients after limited lumbar discectomy: A controlled randomized study of pain response in symptomatic and asymptomatic subjects. Spine 2000: 25: 3065-3071.
156. Fredman B, Nun MB, Zohar E, et al. Epidural steroids for treating "failed back surgery syndrome" is fluoroscopy really necessary? Anesth Analg 1999: 89: 1330-1331.
157. Fibuch EE. Percutaneous epidural neuroplasty: Cutting edge or potentially harmful pain management. Reg Anesth Pain Med 1999: 24: 198-201.
158. Aldrete JA, Zapata JC, Ghaly RF. Arachnoiditis following epidural adhesiolysis with hypertonic saline. Report of two cases. Pain Digest 1996: 368-370.
159. Robertson JT. The rape of the spine. Surg Neurol 1993: P39: 5-12.
160. Myles PS. Editorial: The best evidence comes from large randomized controlled trials. Lancet 1996: 347: 984-5.
161. Heggeness MH, Watters WC, Gray PM. Discography of lumbar discs after surgical treatment for disk herniation. Spine 1997: 22: 1606-1609.
162. Hecht BP, Fischgrund JS, Herkowitz HN, Penman L, Toth JM, Shirkhoda A. The use of recombinant human bone morphogenetic protein 2 (rhBMP-2) to promote spinal fusion in a nonhuman primate anterior interbody fusion model. Spine 1999: 24: 7: 629-636.
163. Stonajovic MP. Stimulation methods for neuropathic pain control. Curr Pain Headache Rev 2004: 5: 6-13.
164. Nerubay J, Urganit B, Bubis JJ, et al. Stimulation of bone formation by electrical current on spinal fusion. Spine 1986: 11: 167-9.
165. Kane WJ. Direct current electrical bone growth stimulation for spinal fusion. Spine 1988. 13: 363-5.
166. Hall BB, Asher MA, Zang RH, Quinn LM. The safety and efficacy of the Isola implant system for the surgical treatment of degenerative disk disease. Spine 1995: 21: 982-94.

9 Figures

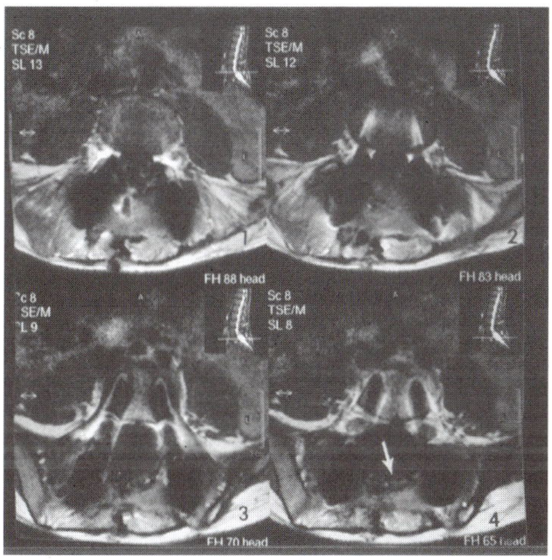

Figure 1: MRI of the Lumbar spine, post fusion with hardware. Notice frames 1 and 2 show the head of the two pedicular screws; in frame 2, clumped nerve roots can be seen within the dural sac. In frame 3 a far too centrally placed screw entered the vertebral canal, deforming the dural sac that developed a pseudomeningocele (small square). Nerve roots are clumped in a "string of pearls" along the posterior wall of an enlarged dural sac (white arrow), frame 4.

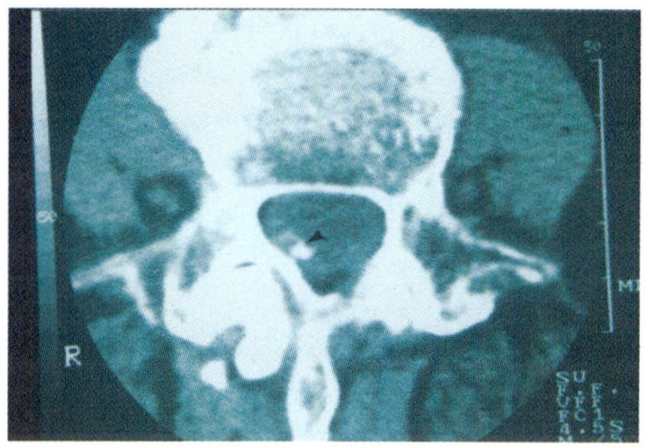

Figure 2: CAT scan of the lumbar spine in a patient with osteoporosis showing a calcification (black arrow) within the right side of the dural sac, taken 14 months after a left laminectomy.

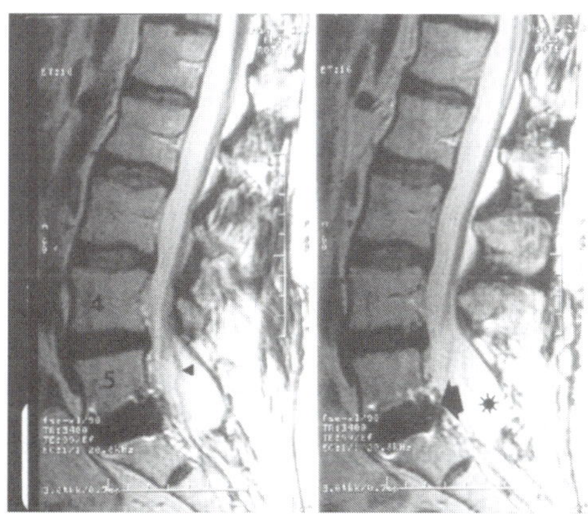

Figure 3: Lumbarization of S1 vertebra noted on both films, after replacement of the L5-S1 disk (large black arrow head), resulting in dural sac ectasia (black asterisk), thickened nerve roots (small black arrow head), arachnoiditis and fibrosis anterior, posterior and inferior from the thecal sac.

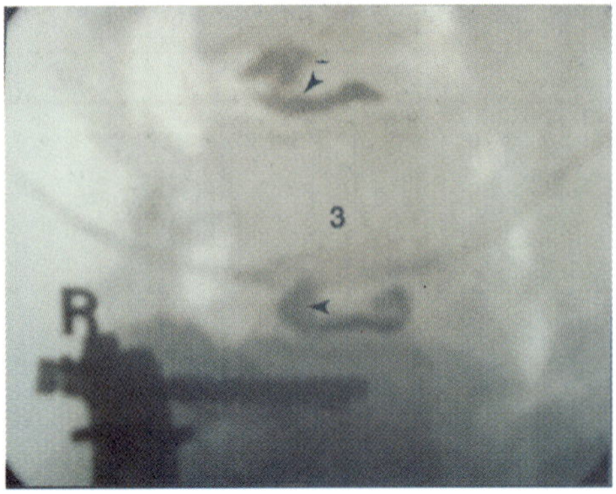

Figure 4: Plain roentgenogram, showing a discogram after having injected contrast media within the L2-L3 and the L3-L4 intervertebral discs.

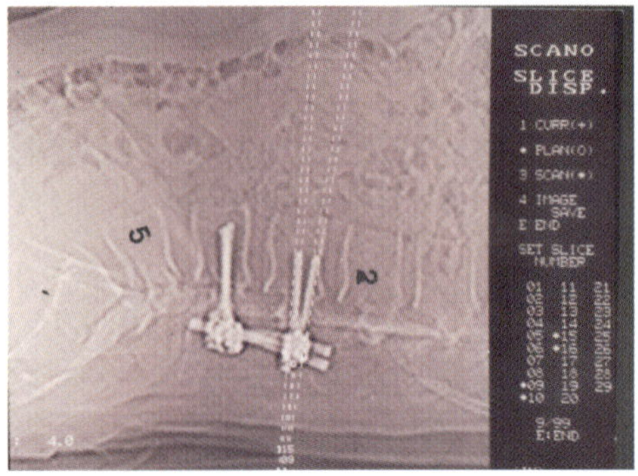

Figure 6: Lumbar spine 3-Dimentional CAT scan, depicting pedicular screws and plates, fusing the L3 and the L4 vertebrae. One of the screws distal tip, is just under the upper plate of L3.

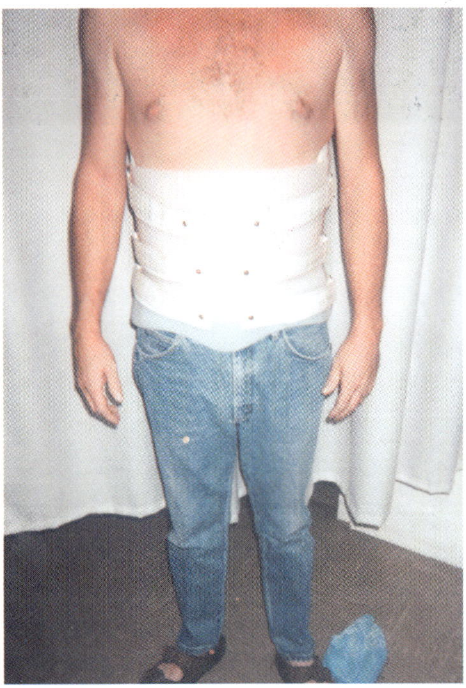

Figure 5: Low thoraco-lumbar-sacral brace.

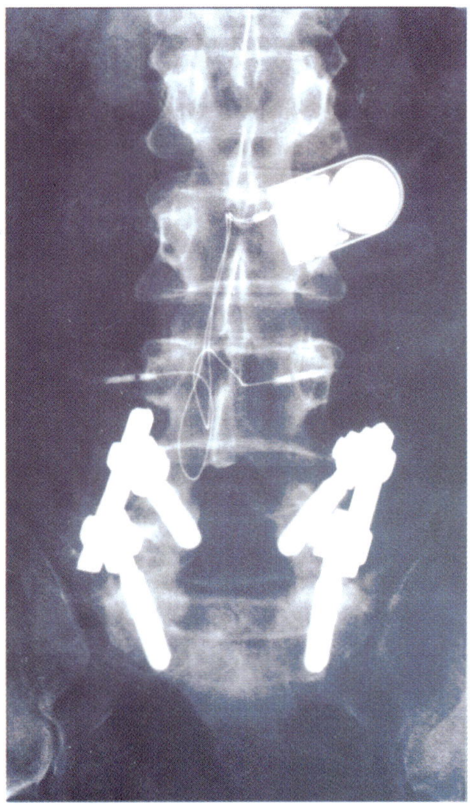

Figure 7: Pedicular screws and vertical bars fusing L5 and S1 vertebrae. Notice the tip of the L5 screws protruding into the vertebral canal and a "bone growth stimulator" at about the level of L3 with the two electrodes located at about the L3-L4 facet joints.

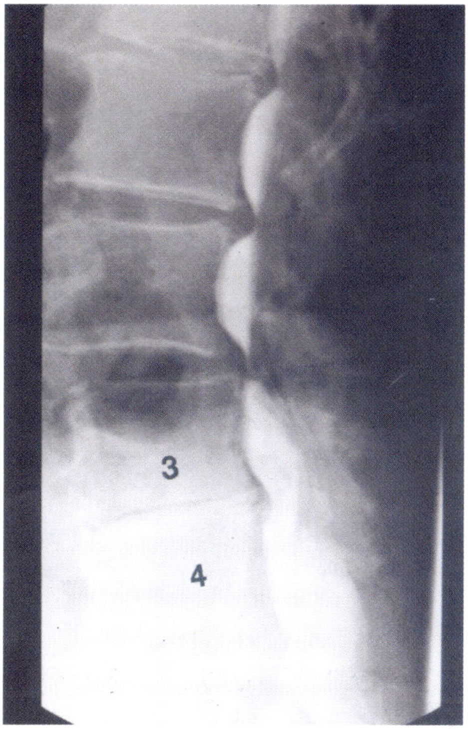

Figure 8: Myelogram of the lumbar spine showing multiple filling defects suggesting protrusion or herniation of the corresponding discs. The L3 and L4 vertebrae are in direct contact (kissing) with complete loss of the intervertebral disk, after a failed fusion.

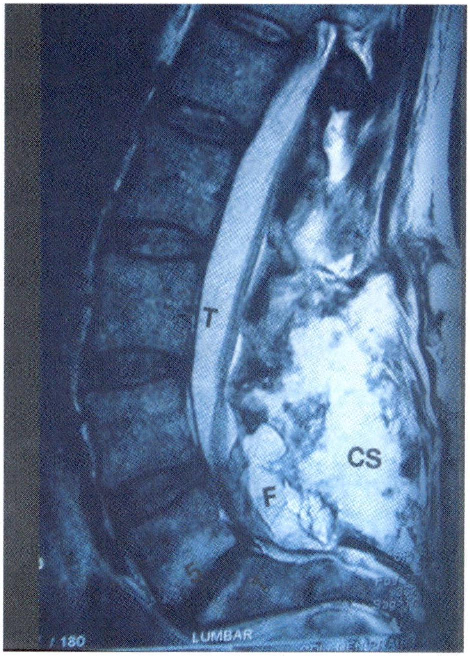

Figure 9: Sagittal view of an MRI of lumbar spine taken three days after a L5-S1 laminectomy at which time a dural tear was produced. The repair included the transfixion of fat (F) tissue, but the leak of CSF (CS) continued after the wound closure then began to exert pressure against the thecal sac (T) and the nerve roots of the cauda equina. The L5-S1 disk is protruding again.

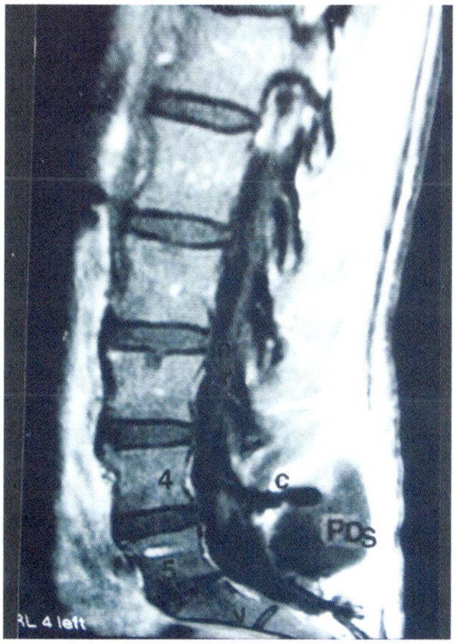

Figure 10: Sagittal view of an MRI of the lumbar spine showing a pseudomeningocele (PDS) still in communication (c) with the thecal sac. A laminectomy and discectomy at L5-S1 produced a marked reduction in the height of the disk.The nerve roots (nr) are thickened. A vestigial S1-S2 (v) disk is noted.

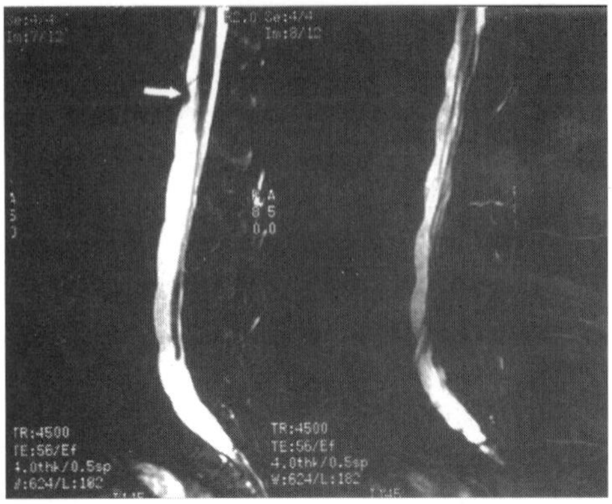

Figure 11: Sagittal view of an MRI of the lumbar spine showing a herniated T12-L1 disk (white arrow), impinging upon the thecal sac and the spinal cord. The distal nerve roots are tethered from L1 to L3.

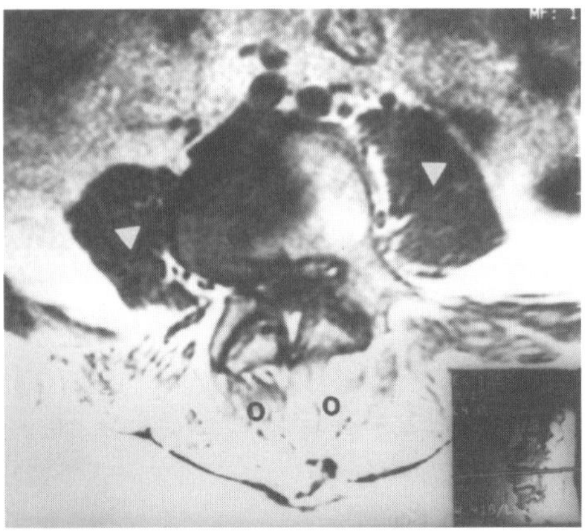

Figure 12: CAT scan of the lumbar spine, showing a stenosis of the vertebral canal with hypertrophic facet joints. Although the spinous process had been removed, the epidural space was retained (white triangle) because the laminotomy was not complete. The posterior paravertebral muscles (o) appear to be atrophic, in comparison to the psoas muscles (white triangles).

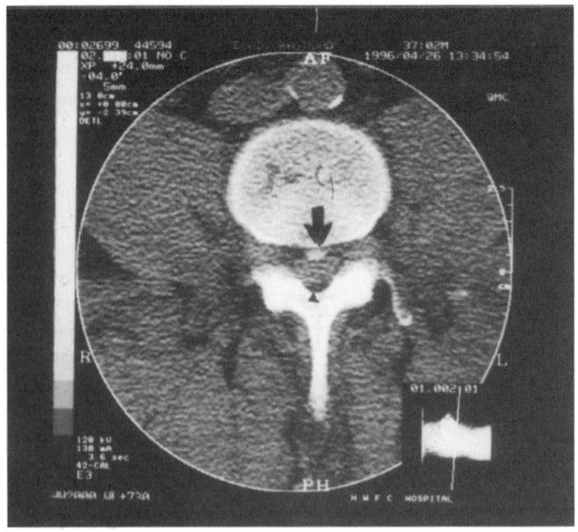

Figure 13: CAT scan of the lumbar spine at the L3-L4 level with a loose fragment of disk (black arrow) after an L2-L3 discectomy. The dural sac was displaced posteriorly with reduction of the posterior epidural space's size (small black arrow).

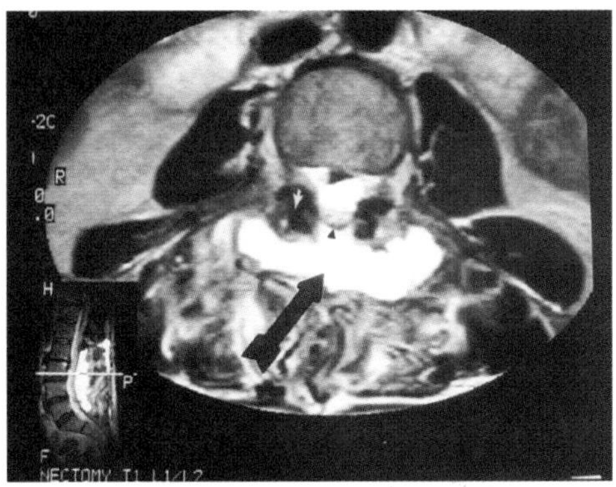

Figure 14: Axial view of an MRI of the lumbar spine demonstrating intrathecal and extradural (large arrow) hematoma, displacing the cauda equina posteriorly (small black arrow). The right facet joint (small white arrow) is shown hypertrophic.

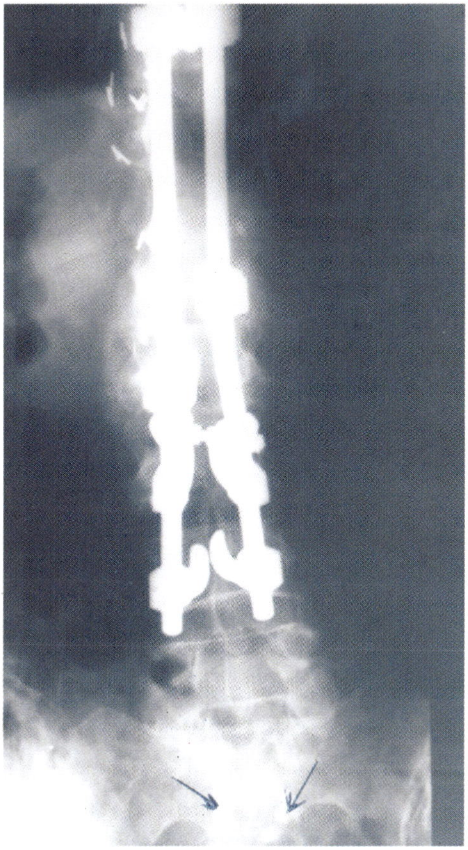

Figure 15: Plain AP film of the thoraco-lumbar spine showing Harrington rods applied to correct scoliosis. Small radicular cysts (arrows) containing pantopaque are shown at the S1, S2, and S3 levels.

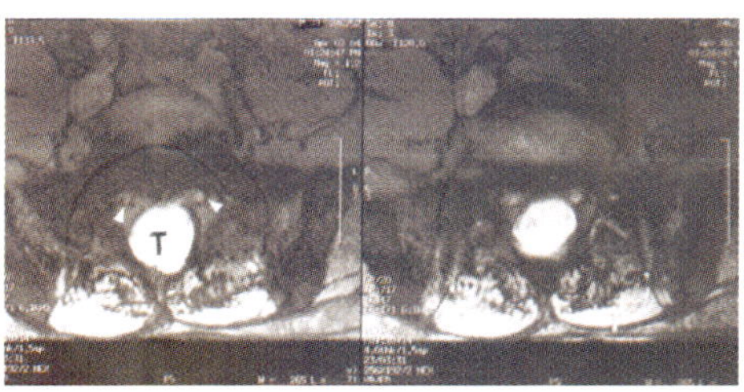

Figure 16: Axial views of an MRI of the L5 vertebra, showing extensive epidural scarring, anterior to the thecal sac (T) that include several asymmetrically situated nerve roots, some of which are adhered to the dural wall. The fibrosis surrounds both S1 nerve roots (white arrows).

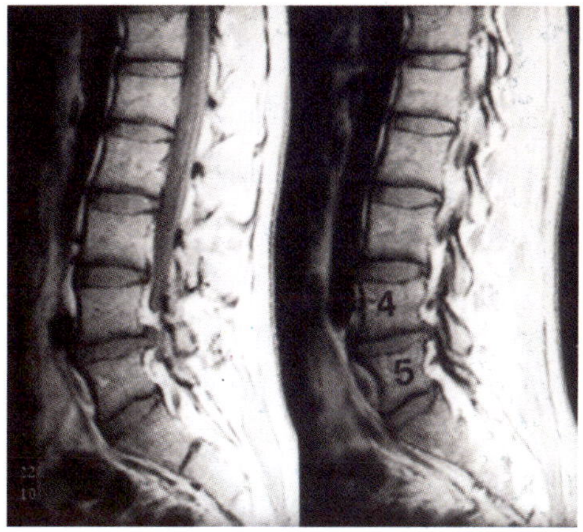

Figure 17: Sagittal views of an MRI of the lumbar spine showing a herniated L4-L5 disk.

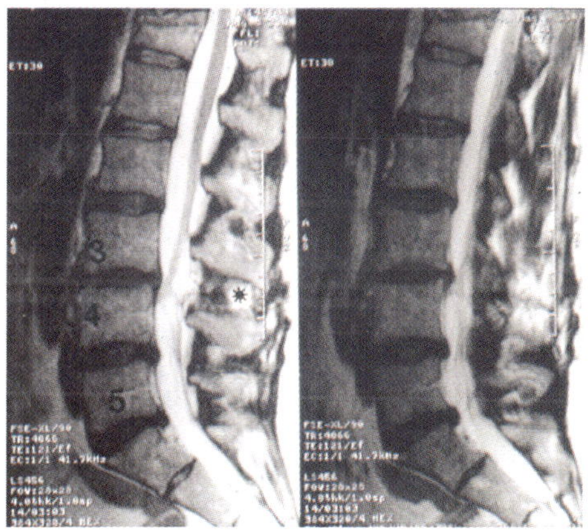

Figure 18: Sagittal view of an MRI of the lumbar spine demonstrating herniated discs at the L3-L4, L4-L5 and L5-S1 levels. The L3-L4 interspinous space has scarring (*) from a previous laminectomy that resulted in arachnoiditis, as demonstrated by the anterior advancement and thickening of the nerve roots, also adhered to the anterior and posterior walls of the thecal sac.

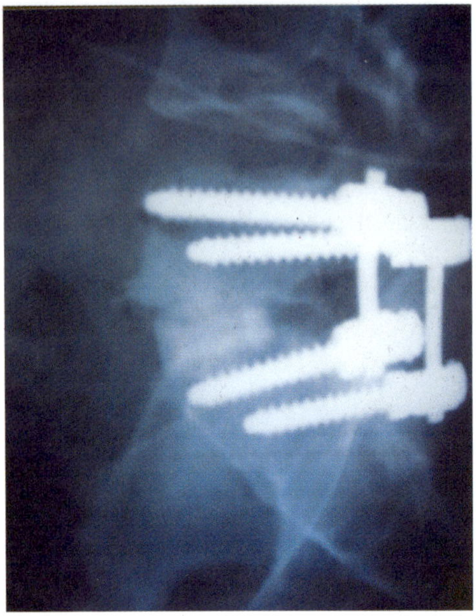

Figure 19: Lateral plain roentgenogram of the lumbar spine showing a too far anteriorly misplaced cage placed in the L5-S1 intervertebral space. One of the pedicular screws' tip protrudes through the anterior plate of the vertebral body.

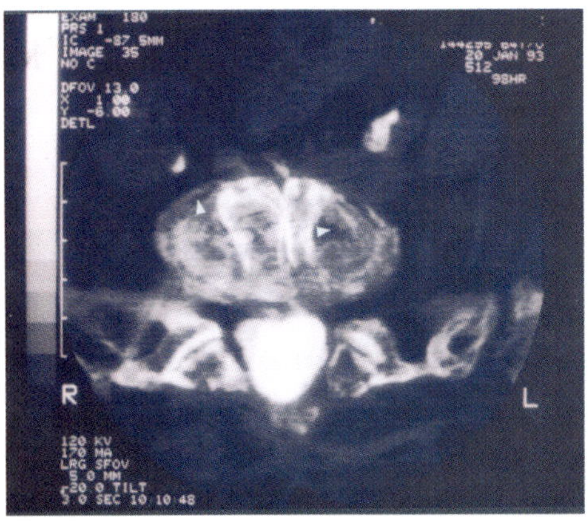

Figure 20: CAT scan of the lumbar spine showing partial arthrodesis between L4-L5 with some "vacuum" areas (white arrow heads); the bone graft leaves have almost been totally integrated into the fusion. The dural sac is dilated, with a clump of nerve roots in the anterior right corner of the sac; multiple small bone fragments are present posterior to the theca. Bilateral spondylosis is also present.

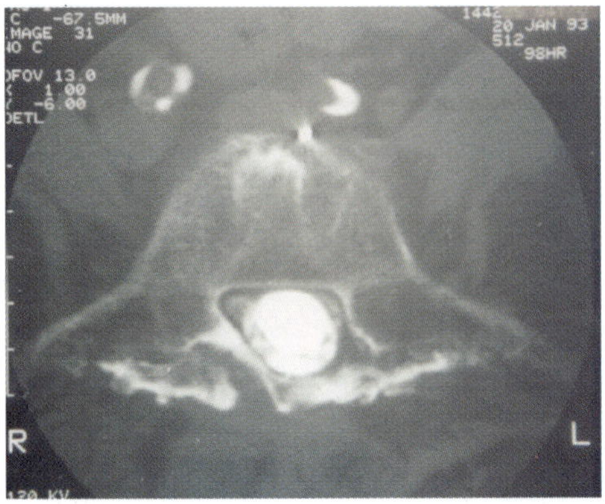

Figure 21: CAT scan of the lumbar spine depicting clumped nerve roots adhered to the wall of the dural sac, which is dilated. After a laminotomy; the left lamina has been substituted by bone growth that extends to the transverse process.

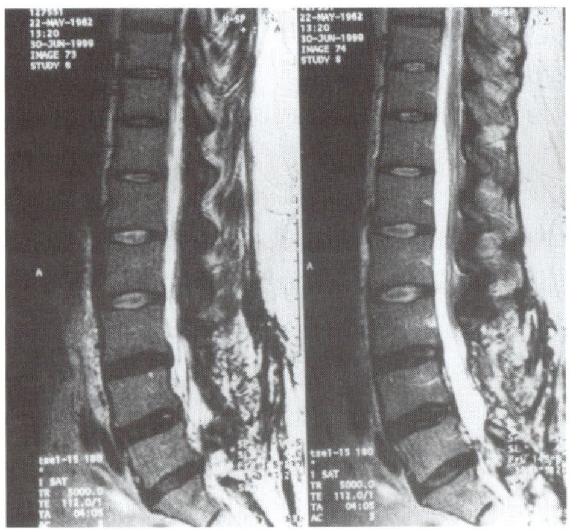

Figure 22: MRI of the lumbar spine showing extensive laminotomies from L3 down to L5 showing considerable peridural scarring and fibrosis mostly posterior to the theca and slight dilatation of the sac. The nerve roots appeared displaced anteriorly on the left frame.

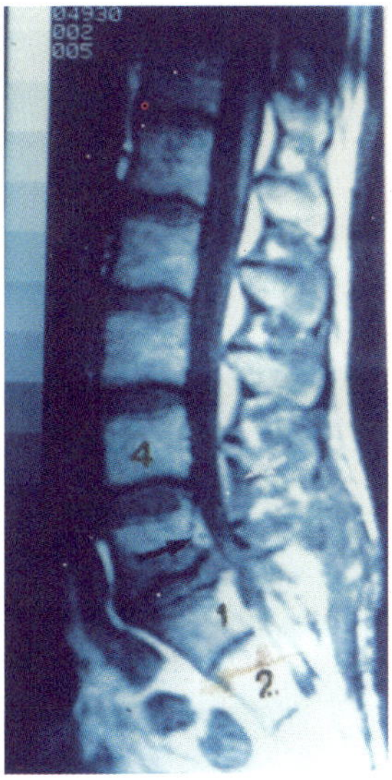

Figure 23: Sagittal view of an MRI of the lumbar spine, showing the inflammatory appearance of discitis (above and below the disk) with a narrow intervertebral line at L5-S1 level. The black arrow points to an epidural abscess surrounding the thecal sac, invading the epidural space at L4-L5 (white arrow) and L5-S1 spaces, extending to the fascia. A vestigial S1-S2 disk is noted.

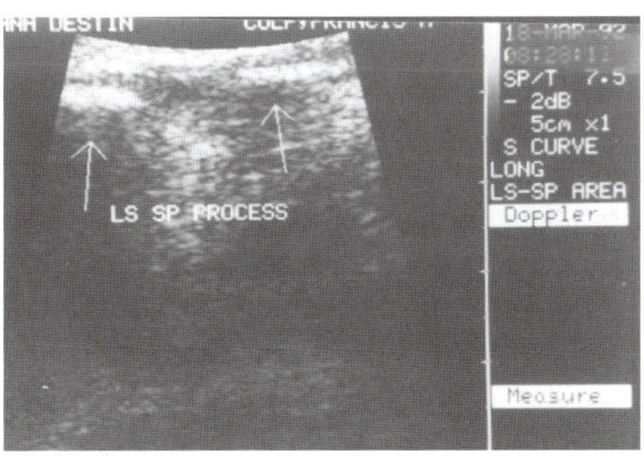

Figure 24: Fascitis between two spinal processes diagnosed by ultrasound.

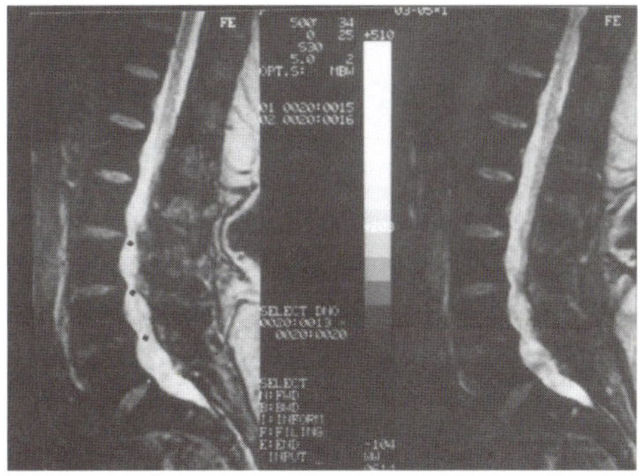

Figure 25: Sagittal view of an MRI of the lumbar spine showing spinal stenosis with narrowing of the vertebral canal (small black diamonds) by a combination of bulging L2-L3, L3-L4 and L4-L5 and hypertrophic facet joints at the L2-L3 and L3-L4 levels.

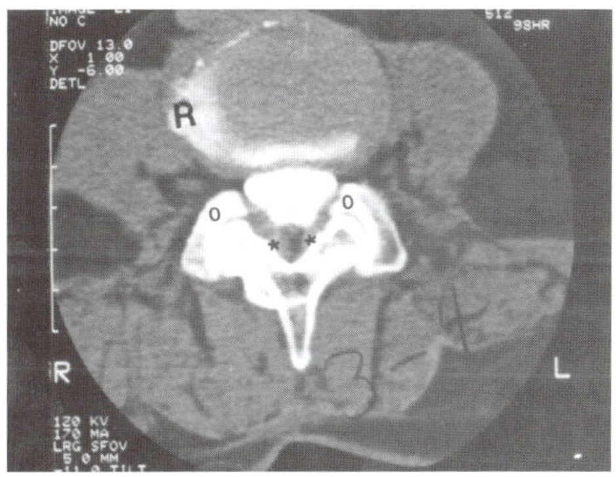

Figure 26: A CAT scan of the lumbar spine after a myelogram showed the L3-L4 disk with right lateral degeneration (R), spinal stenosis from a combination of short pedicles, hypertrophy of the ligamentum flavum (*) and spondylosis (o). The epidural space is narrow.

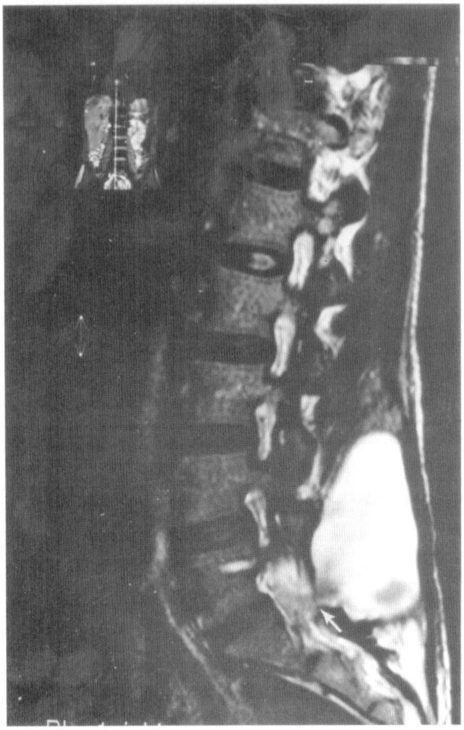

Figure 27: Sagittal view of an MRI of the lumbar spine showing a pseudomeningocele connecting to the subarachnoid space (white arrow) by a small narrow channel (eight weeks after laminectomy and attempted spinal fusion).

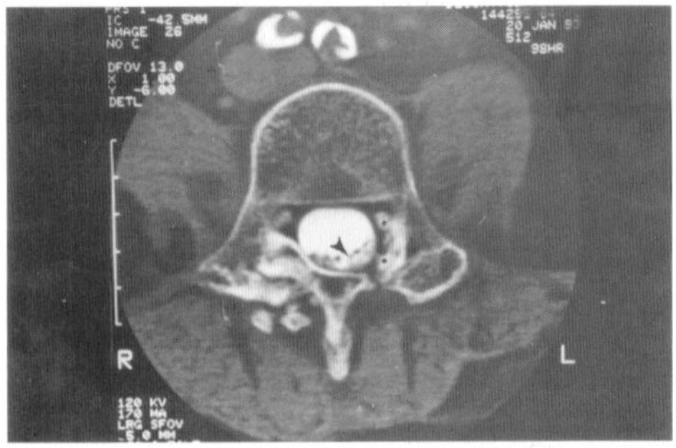

Figure 29: Cat scan of the lumbar spine showing a dilated thecal sac, adhered to the right lamina containing clumped nerve roots (black arrows), mostly on the left side. A prior laminotomy is evident on the left with abundant scarring within the vertebral canal (black diamonds). Loose bone fragments are noted next to an attempted fusion of the right facet joint.

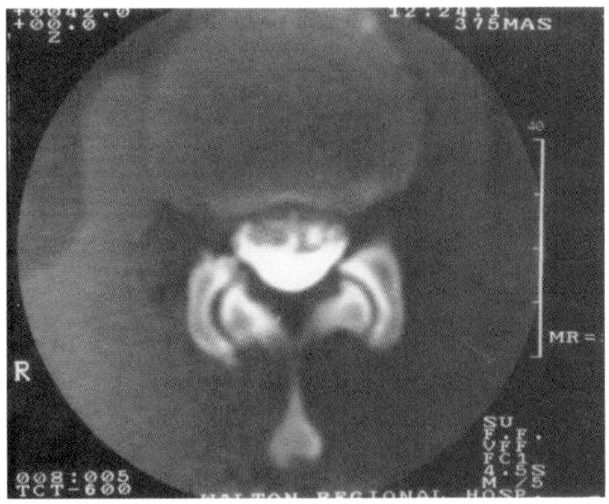

Figure 30: CAT scan of the lumbar spine, post myelogram, showing enlarged, swollen (enhanced) nerve roots located next to the anterior wall of the dural sac.

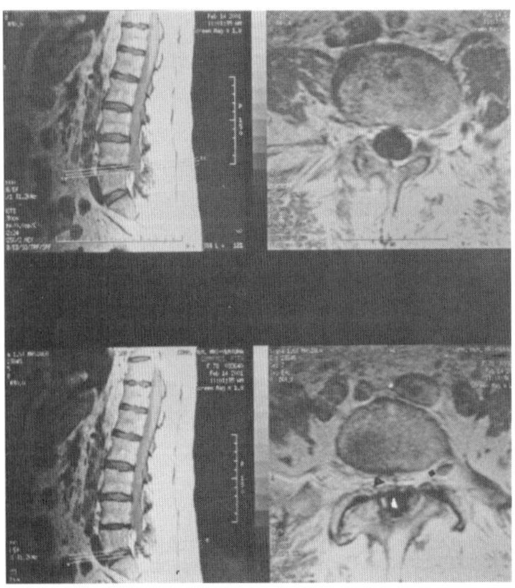

Figure 28: Sagittal and axial views of Lumbar spine MRIs postlaminectomies at L4-L5 (upper frames) showing a "pear-like thecal sac, adhered to the right lamina. The L5-S1 levels (lower frames) demonstrate a narrowed deformed dural sac (small white arrow) displaced posteriorly by fibrosis (black arrow) that have developed posterior to the vertebral body. Only the right nerve root is seen leaving the lateral foramen, because the "cuts" were not made parallel to the disk.

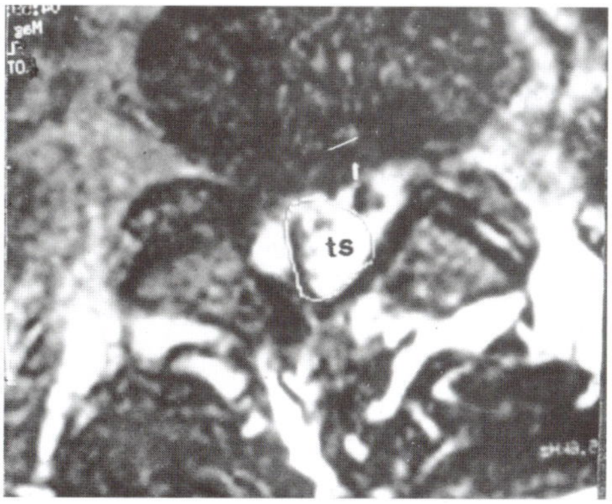

Figure 31: Axial view of an MRI of the lumbar spine showing a post left laminectomy with the nerve roots adhered to the right side of the deformed thecal sac (ts) and a small fragment of calcified disk posterior to the vertebral body. Bilateral spondylosis is also noted.

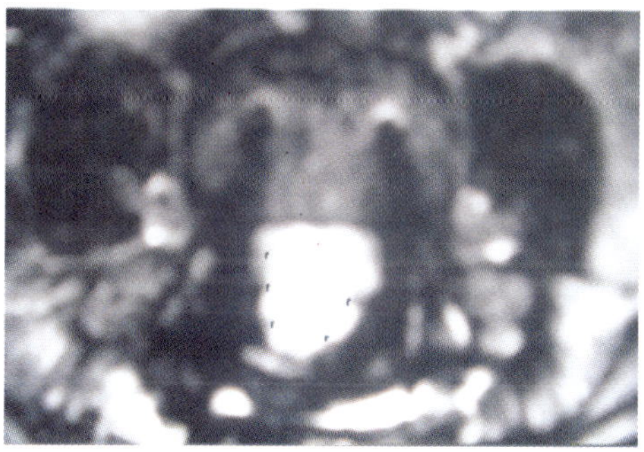

Figure 32: Axial view of an MRI of the lumbar spine showing pedicular screws placed into the L4 vertebra. The thecal sac is dilated and has several nerve roots (r) adhered to its wall.

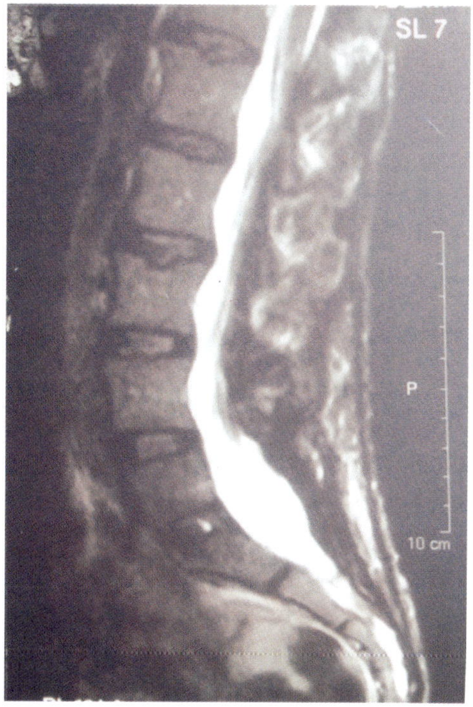

Figure 33: Sagittal view of an MRI of the lumbar spine showing a dilated thecal sac below the L4-L5 disk level, four months after a L5-S1 laminectomy.

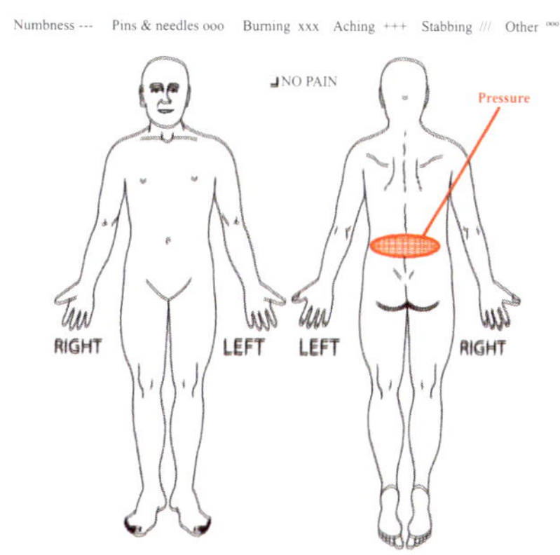

Figure 34: Pain drawing filled by a patient who wrote "pressure" as the main discomfort from a dilated dural sac.

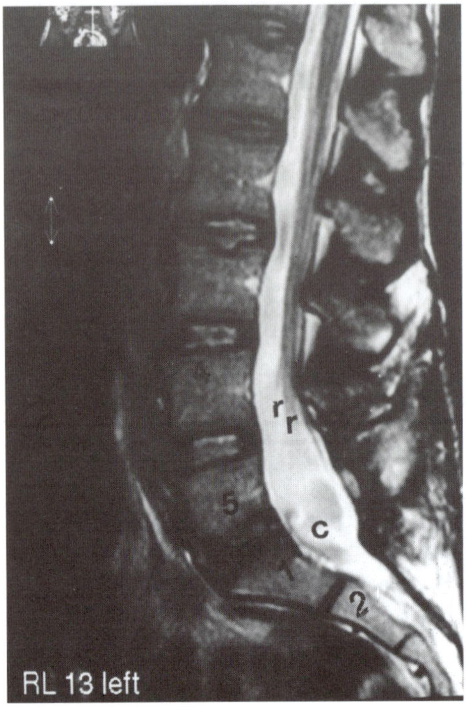

Figure 35: Sagittal view of an MRI of the lumbar spine demonstrating an L5-S1 laminectomy with ample scarring and fibrosis extending from L4 to S2. The dural sac below the L4 vertebra is dilated, with thickened nerve roots (r) and intrathecal pseudocysts (c). There are vestigial discs at S1-S2 and S2-S3. Small posterior epidural spaces are noted at L4-L5 and L5-S1.

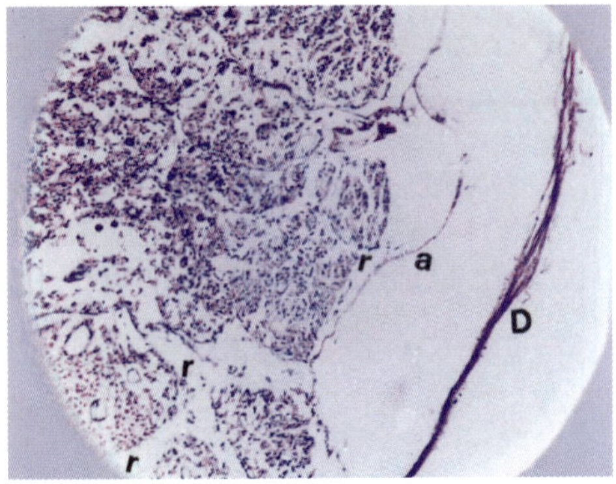

Figure 37: Microscopic (x30) histological section of the thecal sac of a rat that underwent a "sham" laminectomy without damage to the dural wall (D). The nerve roots (r) are clumped and have a geometrical morphology with abnormal distribution of axons. The dural sac was not damaged.

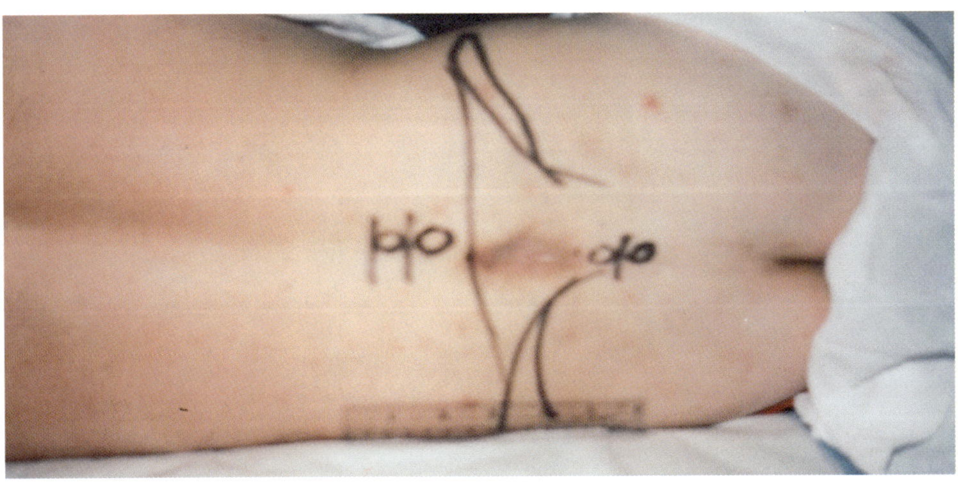

Figure 36: Wide scar from an attempted fusion and laminectomy, four years prior. An epidural abscess and soft tissue infection developed, resulting in removal of the hardware and healing of the wound by second intention. Extensive peridural fibrosis and arachnoiditis occurred, subsequently.

Glossary

10

A

Acute Pain. An unpleasant sensory, perceptual and emotional experience provoked by noxious stimulation produced by injury and/or disease.

Addiction. Psychological, physiological and somatic syndrome overwhelmingly directed toward the use of a drug to experience its effects and to assure its supply.

Analgesia. Absence of pain in response to stimulation that would normally be painful.

Ankylosis. Limitation of the normal movements of a joint.

Arachnoid Cysts. Outpouchings of the arachnoid lining. They are usually considered congenital. If they compress the spinal cord, the cauda equina or individual nerve roots, they can be associated with pain, sensory changes, urinary dysfunction and weakness.

Arachnoiditis. Inflammation of the arachnoid usually brought about by an irritant substance or neural injury within the neuroaxis.

Arachnoradiculitis. Arachnoiditis involving mostly the nerve roots.

ARC. Arachnoiditis.

Arthritis. Joint inflammation often accompanied by pain, swelling, stiffness and deformity.

Arthrodesis. The fusion of two bones.

Atrophy. Reduction in the volume, weight and strength of a contractile organ.

B

Blood-Brain Barrier. Barrier between blood vessels and cerebrospinal fluid-formed vascular epithelium, the ependimum of the ventricles and endothelium of the capillaries.

C

Cauda Equina. The terminal portion of the spinal cord and the spinal nerves below the first lumbar nerve.

Cauda Equina Compression. Often due to neoplasm, but also by lipoma, in spina bifida occulta, constricting fibrous bands or by chronic arachnoiditis (which usually produces burning pain or a sensation of a vice applied to a leg).

Chronic Pain. A persistent pain for longer than two weeks beyond the usual course of an acute disease or a reasonable time for an injury to heal or that is associated with a chronic pathologic process that causes continuous or intermittent pain.

Chronic Pain Syndrome. Encompasses persistent, intractable pain with a variety of symptoms, some of them exaggerated with psychological overtones and abnormal behavior. Acervule, small granuli within the choroid plexus formed of concentric layers perceived at plain sight.

CSF. Cerebro Spinal Fluid

D

Deep venous thrombosis. A blood clot in one or more of the deep veins of the legs (the most common site), or, the veins of arms, pelvis, neck, axilla, or chest. The clot may damage the vein or may embolize to other organs (e.g., the heart or lungs).

Dependence. Altered state induced by the repeated use of a drug requiring its continued use to prevent pain or the symptoms of abstinence.

Depression. Reduction of activity.

Dermatome. The sensory segmental supply to the subcutaneous tissue.

Discectomy. Surgical removal of a herniated intervertebral disk.

Discitis. Inflammation of an intervertebral disk

Drop foot. Plantar flexion of the foot due to injury, paralysis or weakness of the nerves supplying the anterior tibial muscles. It may result in dragging of the foot or toes while walking (L5 nerve root).

Dyesthesia. An unpleasant abnormal sensation, either spontaneous or evoked.

E

Ectacia. Dilatation of any tubular vessel.

Edema. Excessive accumulation of fluid extravasated into the interstitium.

Encephalin. Nitrogenated substance originated in the brain.

Endothelium. A form of squamous epithelium consisting of flat cells that line the blood and lymphatic vessels, the heart and various other body cavities. It is derived from mesoderm. Endothelial cells are metabolically active and produce a number compounds that affect the vascular lumen and platelets.

Epidural Anesthesia. Anesthesia produced by injection of a local anesthetic into the peridural space of the spinal cord.

Epidural Hematoma. Accumulation of blood within the spine but outside of the dural sac.

F

Facetectomy. Surgical removal of the articular facet of a vertebra.

Fascia. A fibrous membrane covering, supporting, and separating muscles (deep fascia), the subcutaneous tissue that connects the skin to the muscles (superficial fascia).

Fasciculation. A small local contraction of muscles, visible through the skin, representing a spontaneous discharge of a number of fibers innervated by a single motor nerve filament. In association with compression of the spinal cord, ventral roots or anterior horns of gray matter, fasciculation of the muscles innervated by the affected segments will occur, along with progressive wasting and weakness.

Fibrosis. Proliferation of fibrous tissue.

Fracture. Interruption of continuity of a bone.

H

HNP. Herniated nucleus pulposus.

Hypertrophy. An increase in the size of an organ or structure, of the body.

I

Inflammation. Morbid complex phenomenon defined as a response by the body against an irritant, infectious or traumatic injury followed by vasoconstriction then vasodilatation, exodus of fluid from the capillaries to the interstitium.

Intrathecal Hematoma. Accumulation of blood inside the dural sac.

Ischemia. Reduction or absence of blood flow.

K

Kyphosis. Abnormal curvature, with dorsal prominence of the spinal column.

L

Laminectomy. The excision of a vertebral posterior arch, usually to remove a lesion or herniated disk.

Leukotriene. Any of a group of arachidonic acid metabolites that functions as a chemical mediator of inflammation.

Lumbarization. Non-fusion of the first sacral vertebra with the sacrum, therefore functioning as an additional (sixth) lumbar vertebra.

Lupus erythematosus (systemic). A chronic autoimmune inflammatory disease involving multiple organ systems and marked by periodic acute episodes. Its name is derived from the characteristic erythematous "butterfly" rash over the nose and cheeks, which resembles a wolf's snout.

M

Meningismus. Irritation of the brain and spinal cord with symptoms simulating meningitis but without actual inflammation.

Morbidity. The number of sick persons or cases of disease in relationship to a specific population.

Morphology. The science of structure and form of organisms without regard to function.

MRI. Magnetic Resonance Imaging

Myelin. White substance surrounding nerve trunks constituted mostly by lipids.

N

Narcotic. A drug that depresses the central nervous system, thus relieving pain and producing sleep. Most narcotics are habit-forming. Excessive doses produced unconsciousness, stupor, coma, respiratory depression, pulmonary edema and sometimes death.

Neuralgia. Paroxysmal pain which extends along the course of one or more nerves. Many varieties are distinguished according to the part affected or the cause.

Neuritis. Inflammation of a nerve or nerves.

Neuroaxis. Spinal cord.

Neurogenic. Originating in the nervous system.

Neurolytics. Substances that functionally and anatomically damage nerve tissue.

Neuropathic. Pertaining to or characterized by neuropathy (usually due to nerve injury).

Neuropathy. A general term denoting functional disturbances and/or pathological changes in the peripheral nervous system (in one nerve, mononeuropathy; in several nerves, mononeuropathy multiplex; if symmetrical and bilateral, polyneuropathy). The etiology may be known as diabetic neuropathy, ischemic neuropathy, traumatic neuropathy or unknown. Encephalopathy and myelopathy are corresponding terms relating to involvement of the brain and spinal cord, respectively.

O

Opiates. Derivatives of opium, usually natural.

Opioids. Synthetic derivatives of opium.

Osteophyte. Bony protrusion that develops in the proximity of an inflamed or frequently traumatized portion of bone

P

Pain. An unpleasant sensory and emotional experience associated with actual or potential tissue damage.

Pain Threshold. The least experience of pain that a subject can recognize.

Pain Tolerance Level. The greatest level of pain that a subject is prepared to tolerate.

Paresthesia. An abnormal painful sensation, whether spontaneous or evoked.

Pedicles. The bony process that projects backward form the body of a vertebra, connecting with the lamina on each side. It forms the root of the vertebral arch.

Peridural. Outside the dura mater of the spinal cord.

Proliferation. Rapid and repeated reproduction of new parts as by cell division. The process or result of rapid reproduction.

Pseudoarthrosis. A false joint.

Pseudomeningocele. A false meningeal sac.

Pulmonary emboli. A mass of undissolved matter present in a blood or lymphatic vessel and brought there by the blood or lymph. Emboli may be solid, liquid, or gaseous. Occlusion of vessels from emboli usually results I the development of infarcts.

R

Radiculalgia. Pain along the distribution of one or more sensory nerve roots.

Radicular. Of or pertaining to a nerve root.

Radiculitis. Inflammation of a nerve root of a spinal nerve, especially that portion of the root which lies between the spinal cord and the intervertebral canal.

Radiculopathy. A disturbance of function or pathologic changes in one or more nerve roots.

Rudimentary. Undeveloped, not fully formed.

S

Sacralization. Fusion of the sacrum and the fifth lumbar vertebra.

Sciatica. Pain emanating from the lower back that is felt along the distribution of the sciatic nerve in the lower extremity. It typically occurs as a result of lumbar disk disease and is felt in the back of the thigh and sometimes in the rest of the lower extremity.

Scoliosis. Abnormal lateral deviation of the spinal column.

Spina bifida cystica. A congential defect in the walls of the spinal canal caused by a lack of union between the laminae of the vertebrae characterized by the presence of a cyst. The lumbar portion is the section chiefly affected. The consequences of this defect may include urinary incontinence, saddle or limb anesthesia, gait disturbances and structural changes in the pelvis.

Spina bifida occulta. A failure of the vertebrae to close, without hernial protrusion.

Spinal Anesthesia. Anesthesia produced by injection of anesthetic into the subarachnoid space of the spinal cord.

Spinal stenosis. A narrowing of the spinal canal caused by degenerative or traumatic changes at the level of the lumbar vertebrae.

Spondylolisthesis. Any forward slipping of one vertebra on the one below it. Predisposing factors include spondylolysis degeneration, elongated pars, elongated pedicles, and birth defects in the spine such as spina bifida..

Spondylolysis. The breaking down of a vertebral structure. Malalignment of the vertebrae.

Spondylosis. Facet joint arthritis or hypertrophy.

Subarachnoid Block (also Spinal Anesthetic or Intrathecal Block). An interruption of the nerve conduction within the arachnoid (intermediate and deep) layers.

Subdural. Beneath the dura mater.

V

Vestigial disk. Rudimentary disk